LEADERS, VISIONARIES, AND DREAMERS

EXTRAORDINARY PEOPLE WITH DYSLEXIA AND OTHER LEARNING DISABILITIES

DISABILITY AND THE DISABLED – ISSUES, LAWS AND PROGRAMS

Additional books in this series can be found on Nova's website under the Series tab.

Additional e-books in this series can be found on Nova's website under the e-book tab.

LEADERS, VISIONARIES, AND DREAMERS

EXTRAORDINARY PEOPLE WITH DYSLEXIA AND OTHER LEARNING DISABILITIES

PAUL J. GERBER, PH.D.

AND

MARSHALL H. RASKIND, PH.D.

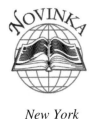

New York

Library of Congress Cataloging-in-Publication Data

ISBN: 978-1-62808-873-1

Published by Nova Science Publishers, Inc. † New York

To Veronica and Tabasco

P.J.G.

To my family – my wife, Lisa, and daughters, Ilana and Emily,
for their endless love, support, and understanding

M.H.R.

CONTENTS

Preface   ix

Acknowledgments   xi

Authors' Note: Defining Our Terms   xiii

Introduction   xv

Chapter 1   Research from the Inside Out   1

Chapter 2   Biographical Sketches   5

Chapter 3   Should "It" Be Called a Learning Disability,
                 Learning Difference, or What?   17

Chapter 4   The Challenges of Learning
                 Disabilities in Adulthood   21

Chapter 5   Recollections of Being a Student   25

Chapter 6   Now and Then   29

Chapter 7   Finding a Niche   33

Chapter 8   Can Dyslexia and Other Learning
                 Disabilities Be Considered a Gift?   39

Chapter 9   Problem-Solving as a Way of Life   45

Chapter 10   Critical Incidents along the Way   49

Chapter 11   Teachers: The Good, the Bad, and the Ugly   55

Chapter 12   Disclosing their Learning Disabilities   59

Chapter 13   Tech Support   **65**

Chapter 14   Sporting Chance   **69**

Chapter 15   Paying it Forward   **73**

Chapter 16   Too Tidy a Tale   **75**

Chapter 17   In Retrospect: Wisdom about
                  their Learning Disabilities   **79**

Epilogue   **85**

Recommended Reading and Works Cited   **87**

About the Authors   **89**

Index   **91**

PREFACE

For some years now we have known that there are people with dyslexia and other learning disabilities who have done extraordinary things in their adult years. It is not uncommon to hear mention of such historical figures as Leonardo da Vinci, Albert Einstein, Hans Christian Andersen, Nelson Rockefeller, and Walt Disney. Although we must be cautious in assuming such individuals did in fact have dyslexia/learning disabilities based on posthumous diagnoses and anecdotal evidence, simply knowing that they *might* have had such difficulties has provided hope, inspiration and motivation to thousands of children, adults and parents. As one adult with learning disabilities told us in an interview, "If Albert Einstein could do it while being learning disabled, I knew I could do it - and I did!"

In addition to those historic figures, each day across the United States extraordinary individuals with learning disabilities are contributing handsomely to the American experience. However, often times their difficulties and struggles are not known to others as a result of the "invisible" nature of their disability. Frequently, there are no obvious signs that would even hint at limitations or challenges of any kind.

The extraordinary people profiled in this book are among these individuals. Over the last decade we have witnessed politicians with dyslexia and other learning disabilities emerging onto the national scene. In the 2008 election then U. S. Congressman Kendrick Meek was prominent in the media, commenting on our first African-American President and the new-found strength of the Democratic Party. Gavin Newsom, Mayor of San Francisco, moved on to statewide political office to become the Lieutenant Governor of California. Diane Swonk, one of the nation's foremost business economists, has provided ongoing expert commentary about the troubled United States economy on national television outlets such as Meet the Press, CNN, and Bloomberg Business television. Financier and businessman Charles Schwab, has become a household name with his mantra: "Talk to Chuck".

The national conversation has been enriched by these people as well as others featured in this book. Each of these individuals has become accomplished in their own right. All are experts and are deeply respected by their peers in their respective fields. Their expertise is admired and their opinions are sought after. They are also individuals with dyslexia and other learning disabilities– disabilities that are undeniably part of who they are. Their disabilities have accompanied them on their journey to prominence.

The other prominent people featured in this book have also been contributing to the American scene for quite some time. They are best-selling authors Terry Goodkind and Patricia Polacco, renowned scientists Professor Jack Horner and Dr. Florence Haseltine, internationally acclaimed artist Chuck Close, and political and educational leader Gaston Caperton, professional athlete Neil Smith and award winning actor and director Henry Winkler. In all, the group of 12 individuals covered in this book is extraordinary because they have successfully navigated their personal and professional challenges and have become very accomplished despite the odds. They are leaders, visionaries and dreamers whose stories are both inspirational and fascinating.

Paul J. Gerber
and
Marshall H. Raskind

ACKNOWLEDGMENTS

   With deepest appreciation we acknowledge the Charles and Helen Schwab Foundation for believing in this project and funding this research. And to Charles and Helen Schwab for their years of devotion in helping children with learning problems succeed, not only in school, but in life. We would also like to express our heartfelt gratitude to the Leaders, Visionaries, and Dreamers in this book who graciously shared their stories of struggle and triumph.

Paul J. Gerber
and
Marshall H. Raskind

AUTHORS' NOTE: DEFINING OUR TERMS

There is considerable debate surrounding the various terms used to describe difficulties with learning. Among the terms often used are "learning disabilities," "learning difficulties," learning differences," and "learning problems." The term "dyslexia" is often used to describe a specific learning disability in the area of reading. It is estimated that 80 percent of people with learning disabilities are dyslexic.[1] Arguably, there are philosophical and pragmatic points to support the use of each of these terms. For purposes of this book, we have chosen to primarily use the terms "learning disabilities" and "dyslexia". These terms are grounded in the research literature, and are defined as having a central nervous system or neurobiological basis; the term learning disabilities is specified in federal legislation. According to the National Joint Committee on Learning Disabilities (1990),

> Learning disabilities is a general term that refers to a heterogeneous group of disorders manifested by significant difficulties in the acquisition and use of listening, speaking, reading, writing, reasoning, or mathematical abilities. These disorders are intrinsic to the individual, presumed to be due to central nervous system dysfunction, and may occur across the life span. Problems in self-regulatory behaviors, social perception, and social interaction may exist with learning disabilities but do not by themselves constitute a learning disability. Although learning disabilities may occur concomitantly with other handicapping conditions (for example, sensory impairment, mental retardation, serious emotional disturbance), or with extrinsic influences (such as cultural differences, insufficient or inappropriate instruction), they are not the result of those conditions or influences.

---

[1] Shaywitz, S. (2003). *Overcoming dyslexia*. New York: Vintage books.

The International Dyslexia Association Board and the National Institutes of Health, (2002) define dyslexia as follows:

> Dyslexia is a specific learning disability that is neurological in origin. It is characterized by difficulties with accurate and/or fluent word recognition and by poor spelling and decoding abilities. These difficulties typically result from a deficit in the phonological component of language that is often unexpected in relation to other cognitive abilities and the provision of effective classroom instruction. Secondary consequences may include problems in reading comprehension and reduced reading experience that can impede growth of vocabulary and background knowledge.

We will use these terms along with more generic terms like "learning difficulties" and "learning problems" as appropriate. These various terms will be discussed later in the book from the perspective of the eminent individuals interviewed. It should be noted that the official definitions of learning disabilities and dyslexia do not relate to a specific stage of development. Subsequently, they don't apply specifically to adulthood. The only official stage-specific definition for learning disabilities has been proffered by the Rehabilitation Services Administration (RSA) of the U.S. Department of Education in 1985 which focuses on the area of employment, which is consistent with their mission. Gerber and Reiff in 1993 crafted a learning disabilities definition to describe the many issues embedded in adulthood after completing their seminal study on highly successful adults with learning disabilities. Their definition is well-suited to the 12 individuals who are the focus of this book.

> Learning disabilities in adulthood affect each individual uniquely. For some, difficulties lie in one specific functional area; for others, problems are more global in nature, including social and emotional problems. For many, certain functional areas of adult life are limited compared to other areas. Adults with learning disabilities are of average or above average intelligence, but intelligence oftentimes has no relation to the degree of disability. Learning disabilities persist throughout the life span, with some areas improving and some worsening. Although specific deficits associated with learning disabilities are real and persistent, such deficits do not necessarily preclude achievement, and in some cases, may have a positive relationship to achievement. In almost all cases, learning disabilities necessitate alternative approaches to achieve vocational and personal success.

INTRODUCTION

It was only a half century ago in America when students with dyslexia and other learning disabilities were thought of as being stupid, unmotivated and lazy. In fact, even today many believe people with learning difficulties are only "marginally capable." Despite having at least average, and in some cases superior intelligence, their struggles in school may lower their expectations for attaining success and living productive and satisfying lives.

During this same period, parents wanted to believe well-intentioned pediatricians, teachers, and counselors who assured them, "Don't worry, he will outgrow it." Unfortunately, the conventional wisdom of that era never really came true. Students who had learning disabilities and dyslexia in elementary school, facing myriad academic challenges, continued to experience academic struggles throughout their school years. They did not outgrow their learning disabilities, nor were their problems "fixed" or "cured". Children with learning disabilities grew up to be adults with learning disabilities. Unfortunately, there was so much emphasis on learning disabilities and academic achievement, little attention was paid to the impact of their learning disabilities outside the classroom. In essence, learning disabilities such as dyslexia in adulthood were yet to be discovered or acknowledged. It seemed as if the years after school did not even exist.

There is no longer the belief that learning disabilities affect only children and teens. The study of learning disabilities beyond adolescence now takes its rightful place on the continuum of human development. We know that learning disabilities have major implications for adulthood. Moreover, current thinking reflects the wide variety of tasks that today's adults must accomplish every day. No longer is the field of learning disabilities solely focused on academics such as reading, writing and arithmetic; it now also includes a focus on employment, community, relationships with family and friends, daily living chores, and leisure activities.

Amongst the tens of thousands of adults with dyslexia and other learning disabilities, a small number of them have in recent years received notice because of their extraordinary accomplishments. As late as the mid-1980s, success in adulthood had not yet been studied and was rarely talked about. There were only brief anecdotes about becoming highly successful "despite the odds". Moreover, there were posthumous diagnoses proffered by writers that great people in history such as Da Vinci, Einstein, Edison, Churchill and Rockefeller all had learning disabilities. Although many of these claims are unsubstantiated and these presumed diagnoses are still in question today, the focus nevertheless shifted to successful adults with learning disabilities.

In the early 1970s, Harold Baker conducted the first study on successful adults with disabilities, suggesting that individuals with learning disabilities became successful because they had "a fire in their belly." The conclusion was flattering, but not at all helpful in understanding the relationship between success and learning disabilities. Certainly motivation entered into success, but there had to be more. Very little had been written or investigated regarding the notion of success. The field was entrenched in a deficit model, which focused on what such individuals could *not* do rather than what they *could* do. This deficit-driven model was contrary to what many of those in the field already knew that there were Americans with learning disabilities who were doing amazing things despite their difficulties!

Dr. Laura Lehtinen Rogan, a pioneer in the field of learning disabilities, conducted a seminal follow-up study in the mid-1970s that was critical to understanding adult adjustment. This research viewed adults with learning disabilities in a different way; illustrating that subgroups of persons with learning disabilities had differing outcomes; in essence, one size does not fit all. There were those who were highly successful many years into adulthood, others who were moderately successful, and another group who were marginally adjusted to adulthood. For the first time the field was getting a glimpse at the contours of the "learning disabled population" when it grew up.

When Dr. Rogan repeated that study of the same population ten years later, her conclusions were mostly optimistic. The first two groups had virtually conquered the adult challenges of learning disabilities. However, the lowest functioning group was still struggling and had significant difficulties well into their adult years. Her work was continued by Dr. Paul Gerber soon after her follow-up study. The same three groups were found again in another sample of adults ranging from highly successful to marginally adjusted as adults. These studies provided impetus for the field to move on and begin to think and investigate the learning disabled adult population with a differentiated perspective. Subsequently, the segment of the adult population that was the first to receive further in-depth attention and investigation were those given the moniker "highly successful" in the learning disabilities literature.

In the late 1980s, Dr. Gerber investigated a large number of highly successful adults with learning disabilities in order to discover what drove their success. Some of these individuals were high-profile professional scientists, entrepreneurs, bankers, and business people who had achieved notoriety in their fields and were considered exemplars among their peers. Their works included the basic research for high definition television, plots for Academy Award-winning movies, and the development of groundbreaking new products at multinational corporations. All in all, they made a great impact on their communities with their thinking and their action.

This investigation of that highly successful group yielded a research-based model to explain the processes that fostered the successful outcomes described above. All in all, control of one's adult life (every aspect of it) drove the achievement of high success in the population of adults with learning disabilities. However, control was a set of dynamics divided into both internal and external parts. Desire, goal orientation and reframing comprised the internal elements. The external elements identified were persistence, goodness of fit, learned creativity, and use of social supports. Without question there was a coincidence of elements in the model that contributed to success whether from a non-disabled or learning disabled perspective. However, how people with learning disabilities put the model in action from their learning disabled experience made it unique.

When analyzing the phenomenon of success there is no doubt that one has to desire success in order to become successful. It is the unrelenting drive to achieve success that fuels the effort. Moreover, it is desire that helps one to forge on when encountering failure (as is often the case with adults with learning disabilities). While desire is crucial to success it must be directed and focused through goal-setting. Energies expended to work for successful adjustment needs short, intermediate and long term planning. Goals set the framework for accomplishment. So too, they provide a standard for success and failure needed to plan and take the next step of achievement. The process of reframing makes the model learning disabilities-specific. In essence, reframing is re-interpreting the LD experience as a positive one, celebrating strengths, while knowing full well one's weaknesses. Successful reframing allows for the possibility of accomplishment and also links to all the external elements of the model for success. Moreover, reframing has stages of its own. They are: first acknowledging that the learning disability is real and has its specific challenges; second, understanding one's own learning disabilities profile; third, accepting all of the dimensions of the learning disability; and last, planning for functioning in the variety of adult domains while fully accounting for the learning disability itself.

The external elements of the Gerber model emphasize that a person with learning disabilities must interact and adapt to his surroundings in a productive manner in order to maintain the control that fosters success. Persistence underpins the sustained effort to be successful with a kind of "stick-with-it-ness" that is characterized by doing all that needs to be done to be prepared. Goodness of fit links to reframing, essentially matching one's skills and competencies to the demands of a setting, or "finding one's *niche*". Learned creativity stresses that adaptability to any of the situations an adult with learning disabilities faces has to involve an active problem-solving process. Creative thinking becomes important because when one has a learning disability (and can reframe successfully), he/she either has to adapt to a given situation or make the situation adapt to them (the latter being the source of reasonable accommodation). Last, the element of social ecologies, in essence social support, necessitates the thinking that when one has a learning disability, he/she typically cannot succeed on his/her own. They need to have either formal or natural supports to help them, complement their skills. This acts as a "protective factor" identified as being critical to the concept of human resilience. Protective factors serve to buffer circumstances that would ordinarily lead to behavior with negative outcomes.

It is interesting to note that despite different research participants and methodologies, other studies have found a number of elements (or attributes) that tend to support successful life outcomes similar to those described by Gerber. For example, Dr. Marshall Raskind and colleagues conducted a 20-year study in an attempt to identify the personal characteristics and life situations and experiences that lead to successful life outcomes in people with learning disabilities. Results of the research revealed a set of personal characteristics, attitudes, and behaviors that promoted life success, including self-awareness of their strengths and weakness and the ability to "compartmentalize" their learning difficulties; perseverance in the face of adversity; setting specific yet flexible goals, including a strategy to reach them; and the presence and use of effective social support systems. Dr. Emmy Werner (considered to be the "Mother of Resilience" research) as part of her seminal work on risk and resilience found that the "establishment of realistic educational and vocational plans" and the presence of "supportive adults who fostered trust and acted as gatekeepers for the future" were essential components in promoting positive life outcomes for persons with learning disabilities.

None of the individuals included in the research by Drs. Rogan or Gerber had the benefit of the legal provisions and protections of today's federal laws that provide opportunity to Americans with learning disabilities. Laws that mandated fairness in the treatment of persons with disabilities, Section 504 of the Rehabilitation Act of 1973 and the Americans with Disabilities Act of 1990 and its amendments, did not affect them or their success in the least. For the most part, they succeeded via their own devices in spite of the odds. This is also true of the 12 individuals featured in this book.

A somewhat controversial thought in the field of learning disabilities is that "if you have a learning disability, there has never been a better time than today". This statement should not in any way minimize the challenges and struggles of those who have learning disabilities. It just acknowledges the fact that in a previous era there were no mandatory special education laws, individualized education plans, assistive technologies, etc. It simply was a very different time, when even the term "learning disabilities" was being debated amongst professionals across the country. When it came to the issue of adults with learning disabilities, there was even a time (in the early 1980s) when the fundamental question, "Is there such a thing found in adulthood that can be called learning disabilities?" was never asked. Soon to follow was, "What are the chances of them having a successful career." Thankfully, those days are gone, and not a moment too soon.

Part of the conversation that has led to a focus on adults with learning disabilities has been individuals identified with learning disabilities who have served as role models by accomplishing extraordinary things in their respective fields. They are impressive examples for all who face the challenges of learning disabilities. A field that has been traditionally deficit-oriented now has concrete evidence that it is possible to succeed despite a learning problem and, in some cases, succeed handsomely. Our message to children with learning disabilities and their parents, teachers and assorted professionals who work in the field is this: **Dyslexia and other learning disabilities, and success, are not mutually exclusive.** The following research on these extraordinary people serves as ample evidence.

Chapter 1

RESEARCH FROM THE INSIDE OUT

There have been numerous efforts in past years to highlight the successes of adults with learning disabilities, particularly those who are considered highly successful. Their stories have come in a variety of forms– books, videos, articles in the popular press, and first person accounts. Without question they are riveting descriptions of living successfully with the daily challenges of learning disabilities.

This book, however, takes a different approach from others that have tackled success and learning disabilities. It presents the work thematically, unfolding chapter by chapter, and builds upon what we know thus far in an effort to provide and a deeper and richer understanding and greater detail of the accomplishments of 12 extraordinary adults with dyslexia and other learning disabilities.

Each individual in this study had previously been professionally identified as having a learning disability and/or dyslexia. All interviews were conducted in person (except for one by phone) by the authors. The interviews took us to seven states, and at the risk of sounding a bit "star struck", we found them quite exciting. We had the opportunity to meet with financier Charles Schwab in his high rise private office with views of the San Francisco skyline. We could not help but think about the significant financial/economic decisions made there that affected millions of investors worldwide. Also overlooking San Francisco was the office of then Mayor Gavin Newsom in City Hall. It was thrilling to realize that we were sitting in the office where he researched, reflected upon and made decisions about major political and social issues that not only affected the citizens of one of the US's largest cities, but also groundbreaking policies and legislation that often influenced other cities across the country. Then there was best-selling author Terry Goodkind, far away from the city lights, located in what some may call "the middle of nowhere" in an austere, but breathtaking Southwestern desert. We met in his home, which he had designed with the same limitless imagination and beauty as he had so artfully created in the palaces and magical settings of his novels.

And who couldn't help but be a bit awestruck talking with the "Fonz," the brilliant actor, director and author Henry Winkler? The opportunity to meet with Chuck Close in his New York City NoHo studio was an incredible experience. It was amazing to be surrounded by massive seven foot plus, penetrating, haunting, photo-like portraits with the man who had painted them and is consider one of the greatest American artists of our time.

What can be said to fully describe the experience of interviewing Jack Horner in Missoula's Museum of the Rockies, surrounded by the remains of dinosaurs and the story of their existence eons ago. There was exuberance in the air that day, as he had just returned from Mongolia where he had found 39 baby dinosaur raptors. Yet he made time to tell us his story and convey his passion about past discoveries and his vision for future paleontological investigation.

Kendrick Meek's Congressional office, just next to the U.S. Capitol, was a bustling place, phones ringing and busy staff. He was multitasking before, during, and after the interview, having to speak on the phone to constituents, consult with other members of Congress, and to go to the House floor to vote. The interview (a thorough one despite the multitasking) was an exercise in his commitment to people with learning disabilities for whom he has had a lifelong passion.

Diane Swonk met with us at her "home away from home", Washington, D.C., while at an economic policy meeting. She was the only woman at the meeting, an experience that was not uncommon in her field. Despite being pressed for time, she was extremely gracious and her insights were analytical and insightful. We sensed that this was the same approach she takes when discussing and debating the economic questions of our time.

How could anyone not be impressed with Neil Smith, the former NFL star? He was a mammoth of a man, yet a gentle giant. He had done it all in sports– All-American, NFL Pro-Bowler, and Super Bowl winner. We met him in a Kansas City hotel "where everyone knew his name". While with us he chronicled his life, and even shed tears as he thought about his journey to success and stardom.

Patricia Polacco lives in a fairy tale setting much like the one she writes about in her children's books. Her home in Union City, Michigan exudes the warmth that can be felt in both her writing and illustrations. The interview was set in her historic home just days before Christmas, which provided a fantasy-like setting for our conversation. She spoke as a story teller as well as a crusader, her recollections and wisdom filled with the uniqueness that connects her to her audience.

The doctor was in and not taking any calls. Dr. Florence Haseltine met with us at her home office, just across the Potomac River in Arlington, not far from National Institutes for Health, so she could give us her undivided attention. She spoke with vivid recollection about her journey from being a dyslexic child to becoming a prominent physician who advocates for women's health issues and influences policy from within the federal government.

New York City (at the College Board Offices in Manhattan) was the site of our conversation with Governor Gaston Caperton. From this vantage point he and his organization provide leadership in higher education in the United States and around the world. "Busy but making time" seemed to be the order of the day. His time with us allowed him to step away from the daily issues and routine of his work to reflect on his challenges with dyslexia and his path to success from West Virginia to the "Big Apple".

Our interview questions were open-ended and allowed these prominent individuals to freely answer, expand and elaborate in any way they felt necessary to tell their story. There were no time limits imposed by us, with interviews ranging from 30 to 90 minutes. Interviews were audio-taped and then transcribed word-for-word. The authors later analyzed each interview and collaborated to share ideas, thoughts, commonalties, and themes. Repeated analysis and discussion continued over a period of one year.

Our intent was not to study these extraordinary people, but rather to learn from them. We wanted to hear their stories, ideas, thoughts and opinions –in their own words– rather than impose any preconceived notions or ideas that we may have formed over the years. (Admittedly, this was not always an easy thing to do.) Emphasis was placed on capturing and reporting the "insiders' perspective" and direct quotations are used in this book to verify and elucidate their experience of living and achieving with learning difficulties.

We acknowledge that this group of extraordinary individuals may not be representative of people with learning disabilities as a whole. We purposely sought out prominent, highly successful, extraordinary individuals with learning disabilities to tell us their stories, struggles and triumphs. They offer lessons about courage, perseverance, hope and triumph. Hopefully, these lessons will serve as an inspiration to all in their life journeys to reach their optimal potential and live satisfying, productive and, rewarding lives.

Chapter 2

BIOGRAPHICAL SKETCHES

It goes without saying that the biographical sketches of these highly successful adults with learning disabilities are just thumbnail descriptions of their lives and their extraordinary accomplishments. In each case much more can and has been written about them. After all, they are the epitome of success in their field and in many cases, household names in American culture.

These individuals have achieved success in a variety of professional areas. They are politicians, scientists, artists, writers, athletes, and business executives, illustrating the great variety of vocations found among people with learning disabilities.

GASTON CAPERTON
POLITICIAN, EDUCATIONAL LEADER

Gaston Caperton is a two-term (1989-1997) governor of his home state of West Virginia. After managing his family's bank and mortgage business he won the governorship in his first attempt at running for elected office. Governor Caperton's tenure as governor was noted for his leadership in promoting education, economic development and the arts.

His first priority as governor, however, was education. He headed up the effort to greatly improve the K-12 West Virginia system. He was once a student in that same educational system and had a difficult time because of a learning disability/dyslexia. During his term as governor, eight hundred million dollars was invested in education. As a result of his focus on technology in the classroom, he received national recognition by winning the

Computer World Smithsonian Award. He has been described as a visionary who "fundamentally changing the educational system of the United States." In 1996, he chaired the Democratic Governors Association.

After leaving office, Governor Caperton taught at Harvard University in the John F. Kennedy Institute of Politics. Later he founded and headed the Institute on Education and Government at Columbia University. In July, 1999 he became president and CEO of the College Board, a not-for-profit educational association with a membership of five thousand of the nation's leading schools, colleges and universities. Among its multifaceted activities, it is best known for administering the Scholastic Aptitude Test (SAT) and Advanced Placement Program tests for college-bound students as well as numerous standardized tests for graduate and professional schools. In 2001, *USA Today* gave Governor Caperton the moniker "education crusader" and named him one of the most influential people in America.

CHUCK CLOSE
PHOTOREALIST PAINTER

Chuck Close grew up as an only child in the state of Washington. At age four he knew he wanted to be an artist and soon after his father made him his first easel and bought him a set of oils at Sears. Despite being told that he was dyslexic (translated by many at that time as being lazy and dumb) and not to set his sights on college, he has become one of America's greatest artists. He is known for his large scale portraits as a photorealist painter described by *ARTNews* as one of the 50 most influential people in the art world.

He attended the University of Washington where he majored in art and graduated magna cum laude in 1962. Soon after, he enrolled at Yale University and received a Master's of Fine Arts. Over the past 40 years he has received critical and popular acclaim for his work. He held his first one person show in 1970, soon to be followed by his first exhibit at the prestigious Museum of Modern Art in New York City.

Through the years he has exhibited all over the world. His works are part of the permanent collection of American museums such as the Art Institute of Chicago, the Smithsonian's Hirschhorn Museum, the Metropolitan Museum of Art in New York, and The National Gallery in Washington, D.C. His work appears in museums in Australia, Belgium, Canada, France, and Hungary.

As a leading person in contemporary art for four decades he has "developed a formal analysis and methodological configuration of the human face that has radically changed the definition of modern portraiture." He works from photographic stills to create paintings that appear to be photographic. Some of his pieces have taken up to two years to complete. His work has been described as "ranging from coolly unemotional likenesses of unidentified people to psychologically charged glimpses of well-known artists" such as Roy Lichtenstein and Robert Raushenberg. In 1988 Close suffered a spinal artery collapse and became paralyzed. Since that time he uses a wheel chair and paints with brushes strapped to his wrist. He often uses a fork lift to gain access to parts of his massive portraits.

He has received countless honors for his work, including honorary Doctoral degrees in Fine Art from the University of Massachusetts, Yale University, and Rhode Island School for Design.

TERRY GOODKIND
BEST-SELLING AUTHOR

Terry Goodkind grew up in Omaha, Nebraska and attended public school. Throughout his school-age years, he struggled with dyslexia and found art to be his favorite subject. He briefly attended college but dropped out and worked as a carpenter, violin maker and antiques restorer. Before he was known for his writing he received acclaim for his wildlife and marine paintings. While building his first home in Maine, Goodkind wrote his first novel, the *Wizard's First Rule*, published in 1994. That book launched the beginning of an illustrious career. At that time the rights were sold for six times the price of any fantasy novel. Ultimately, it became an international best seller.

In total Terry Goodkind has written 13 novels and one novella. All but two have made the *New York Times* best sellers list. In 2008 he signed a contract to publish three mainstream novels with G.P. Putnam Publishers. That same year he collaborated with the director of the *Spider Man* movies to create a full series of his work produced by ABC Studios entitled *Legends of the Seeker*. It ran for twenty-two episodes and was renewed for a second season the following year.

When describing his work Goodkind says, "I don't write fantasy. I write stories that have important human themes. They have elements of romance, history, adventure, mystery and philosophy. . . . In my books fantasy is a metaphysical reality that behaves according to the laws of identity." He says his work is influenced greatly by Ayn Rand and by objectivist philosophy.

FLORENCE HASELTINE, M.D., PH.D.
PHYSICIAN AND SCIENTIST

Despite finding school difficult because of a learning disability, Dr. Haseltine rose to become the director of the Center for Population Research at the National Institute for Child Health and Human Development at the National Institutes for Health in Washington, D.C. Her areas of expertise are gynecology, obstetrics and reproductive endocrinology. After earning her Ph.D. in biophysics at Massachusetts Institute for Technology she received her medical education at Albert Einstein School of Medicine of Yeshiva University. Subsequently, she did her residency at Brigham and Women's Hospital (Harvard) and furthered her training through fellowship experiences.

While at Yale where she did research on *in vitro* fertilization, she collaborated with Yvonne Yaw to tell the story of a fictionalized doctor. This resulted in their 1976 novel *Woman Doctor*, which revealed the gender bias in the medical profession against women in the 1960s and 1970s.

In her position, which she has held since 1985, she oversees the basic reproductive health research sponsored by the federal government. In 1995 she founded Haseltine Systems Corporation that designs products for persons with disabilities and holds two patents for her work in that area. In 1990 she founded the Society for the Advancement of Women's Health Research and was editor of its journal. During her distinguished medical career she has received numerous honors and awards. She was elected to the Institute of Medicine, has been given the Weizman Honored Scientist award and was appointed as a Kass Lecturer.

In addition, she is a past winner of the American Women Medical Association Scientists Award. *Prevention Magazine* has made her a "Hall of Fame" honoree, and *Ladies Home Journal* has honored her work as a "Champion of Women's Health". When she was awarded the Kilby Laureates Award in 1998, it read "for quietly changing the course of medical history through her dynamic influence on public policy and funding of medical research to include women in critical clinical trials, saving countless lives in the process."

JACK HORNER
PALEONTOLOGIST

Jack Horner grew up in Shelby, Montana, the perfect place to spark an interest in paleontology and dinosaurs. His father was a partner in a gravel business so Jack was surrounded by rocks in his early years. He often went fossil hunting with his father and found his first dinosaur egg when he was eight years old.

His kindergarten through eighth-grade school years were quite challenging for him because of reading, writing, and mathematics difficulties. He barely graduated from high school. His academic career was saved when a Montana State University geology professor noticed his work on dinosaurs and encouraged him to attend his university. He did attend, only to flunk out and get drafted into the Marines. After his military service he attempted university work again. Although he attended the University of Montana for seven years, he never completed his degree, failing the German language requirement because of difficulties stemming from his dyslexia.

He worked for a brief time at Princeton University's Natural History Museum beginning as a "low level" technician and leaving as a full member of the research faculty without a Ph.D. It was at Princeton where he noticed a catchy poster on dyslexia, followed-up on it, and was soon identified as having a learning disability. While at Princeton in 1976 he made his first significant discovery while doing fieldwork in Montana. He found 15 baby duckbill dinosaur eggs that provided the first evidence that dinosaurs were sociable and nurtured their young in nests; disputing the prevailing evolutionary theory at that time. These were the first dinosaur eggs found in the Western Hemisphere; he named the new genus *Maisaura*, "Good Mother Lizard." Since then, he has named two other species of dinosaurs.

In 1987 he took a faculty position at Montana State University. The previous year he received an honorary doctorate from MSU, the only degree he ever received. Additionally, he won the prestigious MacArthur fellowship, also known as the "genius award" for his ground-breaking work in paleontology.

Horner was a technical advisor to all three of the *Jurassic Park* films. In fact, Steven Spielberg fashioned the character of Dr. Alan Grant after Horner. Currently he is a Regent's Professor of Paleontology at Montana State University, and is Curator of Paleontology at the Museum of the Rockies, which was founded in large part because of Horner's work. He constantly publishes new work in popular and scientific forms, always focusing on his primary research interest– the developmental biology of dinosaurs.

KENDRICK MEEK
POLITICIAN

Kendrick Meek was a democratic United States Congressman from the 17th congressional district of Florida from 2003-2011. He succeeded his mother the Honorable Carrie Meek. Meek was elected four times to his congressional seat and received the Democratic nomination for the U.S. Senate in 2008.

According to Congressman Meek, he found school very difficult because of a learning disability/dyslexia. Despite his difficulties, upon graduating high school he attended Florida A and M University where he was a football star and the founder of the Young Democrats Club on campus. He received his B.S. degree and joined the Florida State Patrol after he left college. He was the first African-American to rise to the rank of captain. One of his assignments was to head the security detail of Lt. Governor Buddy MacKay. This role allowed him to see politics close up, even sitting in on meetings with then Governor Lawton Chiles. Subsequently, he served in the Florida House of Delegates and then the Florida State Senate, each for four years. As a state senator he took on the issue of the "One Florida Plan" to end gender and race preferences in state government. He also led a grass roots effort to reduce class size in Florida's overcrowded public schools.

In the U.S. House of Representatives Congressman Meek was on the influential Ways and Means committee. He also served as one of 12 members of the Congress on the NATO Parliamentary Assembly. Additionally, he was on the Democratic Steering and Policy Committee, the Democratic Black Caucus, and is chairperson of the Board of Directors of the Congressional Black Caucus Foundation.

GAVIN NEWSOM
POLITICIAN, BUSINESS EXECUTIVE

A native Californian, Gavin Newsom grew up in the San Francisco Bay area. After graduating from high school he attended Santa Clara University and earned a B.A. in political science. For a time, he pitched on their baseball team as a scholarship athlete but stopped because of an arm injury. Throughout his educational career he faced challenges because of his learning disabilities in writing, spelling, reading, and math. He credits his disability for "teaching him to apply himself with more focus to develop different skills".

His first job out of college was selling pediatric orthotics, his second doing menial tasks for a real estate company. In 1992 he founded the PlumpJack Wine Shop which he developed into a multi-million dollar business with many locations and 700 employees. In 2002, his business holdings were valued at 6.2 million dollars. Among the many innovative things he did was to give a gift certificate to his staff whose business ideas had failed. He believed, "There can be no success without financial failure."

His life in politics began in 1996 when he was appointed to the San Francisco Parking and Traffic Commission. He was elected its president in 1997. That same year he was appointed to the city Board of Supervisors. He gained notoriety in that position for his support of the Care Not Cash program for homeless people. He also drew a lot of attention through his advocacy for reform of the Municipal Railway.

In 2003 he was elected mayor of San Francisco, the youngest mayor in a hundred years. He was re-elected in 2007 with 72 percent of the vote. He describes himself as "pro-development and for smart growth". In 2012 he was elected Lieutenant Governor of the state of California.

PATRICIA POLACCO
CHILDREN'S AUTHOR AND ILLUSTRATOR

Patricia Polacco was born in Lansing, Michigan to Russian and Ukrainian parents. After her parents divorced she lived in Oakland, California for 37 years before moving back to Michigan. While in junior high school her teacher told her she might be dyslexic. She tells this story in one of her books, *Thank You Mr. Falker*. Despite not learning to read until age 14, she went on to study fine art in her undergraduate college years. Eventually, she earned a Ph. D. in art history. At one time she restored pieces for art museums. It was not until the age of 41 that she began to write and illustrate children's books. She had always had talent for illustration, the story writing part of her work came later. Her storytelling ability was cultivated by listening to rich and colorful stories from her elders, particularly her grandmother.

She moved back to Michigan and currently lives in a house on a farm built in 1859 that is thought to have been visited by Abraham Lincoln. It is there that she writes and illustrates her books. She frequently opens her house to the community for storytelling, festivals, literature conferences and charity events.

Her inspirations are many, including Beatrix Potter and the Brothers Grimm. A favorite picture book among many is *The Tall Mother Goose* by Fedor Rojanski. Her artistic hero is Norman Rockwell. Her readers sense her passion as she "weaves lessons from her past into stories for future generations."

Polacco has received numerous awards for her work. In 1989 she received the highest award from the International Reading Association, and in 1992 she garnered an award from the Society of Children's Book Writers and Illustrators. She also won the Golden Kite Award for Illustration and Parents Choice honors in 1991, 1997, and 1998.

CHARLES SCHWAB
FINANCIER AND PHILANTHROPIST

As a young child growing up in California Charles Schwab learned a lot about business from his first jobs sacking and selling walnuts and selling chickens and eggs. It was basic training for what would become a storied career in the world of finance. He attended Catholic school where he struggled with reading and writing, despite showing talent in mathematics, science and athletics. It was not until the age of forty that he found out he was dyslexic after his son was identified as having learning disabilities.

Charles Schwab attended Stanford University and received a B.A. in Economics in 1959. He continued his studies at Stanford, and in 1961 he earned an M.B.A in the Graduate School of Business despite having severe challenges in English and French courses.

In 1971 he founded Charles Schwab brokerage based in San Francisco. Not long after he changed his thinking and his business model to become a pioneer in the discount brokerage business. Over the years he grew his business to nineteen thousand employees and eight million clients with approximately one trillion, two hundred million dollars in assets.

In 1997 *Forbes* magazine called him "the King of Online Brokers". *Business Week* identified him as one of the top twenty-five managers of the Year in 2001. Along the way Schwab has amassed a fortune through his business acumen. In 2012, *Forbes* listed him as number one hundred and four on their list of "Richest People in American" with personal wealth totaling 3.7 billion dollars. He has been Chairman and a director of The Charles Schwab Corporation since its incorporation in 1986. Mr. Schwab is also Chairman of Charles Schwab & Co., Inc. and Charles Schwab Bank, and a trustee of The Charles Schwab Family of Funds, Schwab Investments, Schwab Capital Trust and Schwab Annuity Portfolios, all registered investment companies.

Along with his wife Helen, he is the co-founder and chairman of the Charles and Helen Schwab Foundation, a private foundation that supports entrepreneurial organizations working in education, poverty prevention, human services and health. For years, the Foundation operated a program that advanced and disseminated knowledge and information about learning and attention problems.

NEIL SMITH
PRO FOOTBALL PLAYER, SPORTS EXECUTIVE

Neil Smith left his native New Orleans to begin his illustrious career in football at the national power house University of Nebraska. After winning accolades for his play on defense he was a first round draft choice of the Kansas City Chiefs where he played from 1988-1996. Subsequently he played for the Denver Broncos and in his final season was a member of the San Diego Chargers. While with the Broncos he was on two Super Bowl teams. He was considered to be a very skilled and tough defensive player standing six foot four, and weighing 260 pounds, and having a seven foot one, and one and a half inch arm span.

He is a former owner and executive of the Kansas City Brigade of the Arena Football League which moved from New Orleans (as the New Orleans VooDoo) in 2006 after Hurricane Katrina. He is currently very active in the Third and Long Foundation, founded by his good friend and teammate Derrick Thomas, a member of the Pro Football Hall of Fame. Neil Smith has carried on the work of the foundation since Derrick Thomas was killed in a car accident in 1999. The foundation serves inner city children in the Kansas City area to improve reading and to support those with learning problems– those experiencing the same "frustrations" he had as a student with a learning disability.

DIANE SWONK
BUSINESS ECONOMIST

Diane Swonk is one of the most influential business economists in the U.S., quoted often in the national and international print and electronic press. She is an only child who grew up in the Detroit area, surrounded by the automobile industry and all its associated activities. Throughout her early school years she was told that she was lazy, felt different and hid the fact that she had dyslexia. Regardless, she went on to attend the University of Michigan and received a bachelor's and master's degree there. Her first economics course was taken "on a lark" but she soon found out it was second nature to her. She went on for further study and earned a MBA from the University of Chicago.

She rose through the ranks at Bank One Corporation over nineteen years to become their Director of Economics and Senior Vice President. Since leaving Bank One she has served as a senior managing director at Mesirow Financial in Chicago.

In the Chicago area she is well known for her professional and avocational work. The *Chicago Sun-Times* has called her "one of the most influential women in business in Chicago". She is very well-known and influential on the national scene. She has been an advisor to the Federal Reserve Bank and its regional banks. Also, she has been appointed and re-appointed to the Congressional Budget Office's panel of economic advisors. She is a fellow of the National Association of Business Economists and was its first woman president. One of her predecessors in that role was Alan Greenspan. The *Wall Street Journal* has named her one of the top business forecasters. In her own words she states that she "continues to dedicate much of her time to improving the quality and timeliness of economic data that is critical to policymaking." Most recently, she authored the book, *The Passionate Economist: Finding the Power and Humanity Behind the Numbers.*

HENRY WINKLER
ACTOR, DIRECTOR, PRODUCER, AUTHOR

Henry Winkler was born in New York City to German immigrants. His father was a lumber executive. He received his undergraduate degree at Emerson College in 1967 and a Master's of Fine Arts in drama at Yale

University. After doing commercial work he was cast as Arthur Herbert Fonzarelli, the iconic "Fonz," in the 1970s hit show *Happy Days* by television producer Garry Marshall. Winkler lamented later about that role, "The Fonz was everybody I wasn't. He was everybody I wanted to be." He attributes much of his lack of self-confidence to his struggles with dyslexia.

After *Happy Days* he began his career in producing and directing founding the company Winkler-Rich Productions. He directed television shows such as *MacGyver, Mr. Sunshine,* and *Hollywood Squares* from 2002 - 2004. He also directed movies with such stars as Billy Crystal and Burt Reynolds. He co-starred with Kathryn Hepburn in her last movie made for television, *One Christmas.*

Winkler's movie roles include *Scream* (1996), *The Waterboy* (1998), *Little Nicky* (2000), *Click* (2006), and *You Don't Mess with the Zohan* (2008). He also appeared as the incompetent lawyer on the television show *Arrested Development.* Dating back to the 1970s Henry Winkler has won a bevy of show business awards. In 1976 and 1977 he won the Golden Globe award as best actor for "Happy Days". He was nominated in the best actor category in 1978 and 1979 for Happy Days as well. Moreover, he was nominated three times for prime time Emmys in 1976, 1979 and 1997. In total his filmography lists twenty-eight works from *Crazy Joe* in 1974 to *Sit Down, Shut Up* in 2009.

Over the last decade he has authored a series of critically-acclaimed books (*Hank Zipzer*) which follows the everyday adventures of a bright boy with learning challenges. Henry Winkler also does a great deal of charity work. He has been active for causes such as cerebral palsy, epilepsy, Toys for Tots and Special Olympics.

Chapter 3

SHOULD "IT" BE CALLED A LEARNING DISABILITY, LEARNING DIFFERENCE, OR WHAT?

If you learn differently . . . it doesn't mean you can't learn.
— Charles Schwab, Financier and Philanthropist

"Learning disabilities" is the common moniker currently used in research literature, disability legislation, educational settings and popular conversation. Historically, it is a label that is surrounded by a lot of controversy, even though it has now been used for about four decades. The term "dyslexia" has also been in use for quite some time. It is considered a subtype under the umbrella term of learning disabilities and refers specifically to difficulties in reading. According to the National Institutes of Health, approximately 80% of people with learning disabilities have reading problems.

Another term, which has gained considerable popularity in recent years, is "learning difference" which emphasizes diversity rather than disability. The use of this term raises philosophical and pragmatic questions. For example, what are the implications of the term learning differences regarding legal protections, services, and funding? How does it affect the self-concept of those who experience these difficulties, as well as the perceptions of others? Again, our purpose here is not to offer our interpretation, opinion or understanding of these terms, but rather, to share the thoughts and views of some extraordinary individuals who have lived the experience. So while debate may continue over the most appropriate terms, the goal of our research was to discover, from the "insiders'" point of view, the terms they themselves use to describe their learning issues, the reasons behind these choices, and how their successes may color the use of different terms.

During our conversations with these extraordinarily successful individuals, they referred to their difficulties with a variety of terms including "learning disability," "learning challenge," "learning difference," and "dyslexia." Gaston Caperton referred to both "having a learning disability" and "having dyslexia." Similarly, Dr. Haseltine speaks of "my learning disability," but also mentions her "dyslexia." Terry Goodkind states that "my problem is dyslexia" and does make reference to "disability." None of these four individuals used the terms "learning difference" or "learning challenged." Only Neil Smith exclusively used the term "learning disability." Although, Congressman Meek comments that "his disability is dyslexia," he also frequently referred to "learning differences." Henry Winkler never uses the term "learning disability," but rather references "dyslexia" and "learning challenge." Although there was no interview question that directly asked for their thoughts on the most appropriate terms, several of these adults did provide additional commentary. Charles Schwab says that he prefers to call it a "learning difference" because he "thinks differently." To a lesser extent he thinks that learning difficulty is also acceptable. He goes on to say, "If you learn differently . . . it doesn't mean you can't learn..." Patricia Polacco agrees with the term "learning different." She adds, "I would say learning different, but very different. It's just a different way, it doesn't mean it is right or wrong." Diane Swonk agrees with Polacco, and says, "I call them learning differences. I think differently. The reality is you can be smart and be an idiot, but you can be smart and think differently." Jack Horner also agrees with the term "learning difference." "I do not think of it as a learning disability, not a learning problem. I call it a 'learning difference'." He then goes on to take on the imprecision of the term "learning disability." "You know I am a scientist. I am really into definitions. People use words loosely. Without definitions I haven't a clue what they mean. What dyslexia is to you may be different to me."

On the other hand, it is exactly this imprecision that Chuck Close likes. "I would never use the term 'learning different'. No one expects artists to know anything. So I don't have trouble with it. I think it is somewhat of an advantage in some ways with the term 'learning disabilities' in not being pigeonholed." In essence, the "looseness" of the term allows for more flexibility in interpreting of what "it" is and how "it" manifests in daily functioning. As can be seen from these statements, a variety of terms are used to describe the issues these extraordinary individuals face. While some used various terms interchangeably (e.g., learning disabilities and dyslexia), others seem to prefer using one over another (e.g., dyslexia). In some instances, interviewees stressed their preference for the term "learning difference" which emphasizes a different way of thinking or approaching learning rather than emphasizing a disability or inability to learn. Similarly, "dyslexia" was used by some interviewees to describe difficulties specifically in the area of reading, rather than a more generalized problem or inability to learn. It seems fair to say that each and every one of these individuals was capable of learning and that they were, in fact, extraordinary "learners" albeit with diverse approaches that did not always match or mesh with conventional methods or strategies. For some, the use of specific terms seemed to be a philosophical and emotionally-charged issue, while for others it did not emerge as a critical concern. That is not to say, however, that learning disabilities or dyslexia have not profoundly affected their lives.

It is not possible to precisely determine why each individual preferred certain terms over others, nor is that one of the goals of this study. However, it does not seem to be too far of a stretch to conjecture that the choice of specific terms is a function of each person's specific difficulties, life experiences, background, personality, and world view. And, perhaps with this in mind, we can come to understand that one term does not fit in all cases, again emphasizing the diversity of this group and reminding ourselves that people with "learning issues" represent a highly heterogeneous group, and are not all alike.

So then what should "it" be called? We are not sure that there is a definitive answer to this question-- at least, based on the interviews conducted in this study. On the one hand we might conclude that it should be called anything anyone with such issues wants it to be called. They are the "insiders" living with it, and who better to say what it should be called? At the same time it is important to emphasize that the choice of terms does have some practical implications. For example, "learning difference" has some definite philosophical implications as it emphasizes differences and diversity in learning and recognizes that we are all unique individuals. However, unlike "learning disabilities", this term is not used in federal legislation and it is "learning disability" that provides services, protections and funding for those experiencing learning problems with a neurobiological basis. As, Dr. Sheldon Horowitz of the National Center for Learning Disabilities has stressed,

Learning differences refers to the unique qualities, characteristics and preferences that defines each of us as learners and this diversity in style and

approach is something to be celebrated. In contrast, learning disabilities are
not cause for celebration. They are barriers to success that, once understood
and addressed, can enable individuals to compete, succeed and even excel in
the face of challenges that are often hard to define and that change in focus
and intensity across the lifespan. Federal law recognizes 'disabilities' (not
'differences'), and the language we use to both identify these individuals and
classify their struggles are important. Learning disabilities are not who you
are, it's what you have, and invoking the language of the law enables these
individuals to access services and supports and benefit from protections that
ensure the greatest opportunity for each to reach their full potential.

The debate over the correct term will likely continue for some time. In
fact, it is likely to continue indefinitely considering the meaning, interpretation
and implications of each term relative to specific individuals, settings and
objectives. Nonetheless, it is hoped that the insiders' view of these terms will
help others understand that "one size may not fit all."

Chapter 4

THE CHALLENGES OF LEARNING DISABILITIES IN ADULTHOOD

*I am a dyslexic economist. I don't like to say too many numbers because if the
Fed Funds rate is 1.4, 4.0 or.40 you can flip those numbers. I often say my
favorite quarter is one where growth is 3.3 per cent because I can't mess up.*
— Diane Swonk, Business Economist

Learning disabilities are usually associated with the challenges of
academics during the school years. Reading and writing are known to be
challenging throughout entire school careers. Difficulties in other areas such as
attention, listening, memory, organization and cognitive processing are also
frequently noted. A strict focus on school and academics can obscure an
understanding of what adults with learning disabilities face each day of their
lives. There is no doubt that some of the same issues that confronted academic
achievement and performance in school carry over to adulthood. However,
learning disabilities present themselves in a variety of adult situations such as:
daily living tasks, employment, family, recreation and leisure, and social
relationships. Adults with learning disabilities often encounter daily challenges
in these areas. The extraordinary adults in this book are no different.

Reading still presents problems for most of the adults in this study. Gaston
Caperton exclaimed, "I'm still dyslexic today. Being dyslexic is a nuisance. I
don't like to read speeches. It's kind of an inconvenience and sometimes it
takes me a lot longer to prepare than most people. I have to read it over and
over many times so I'm comfortable with it psychologically". However, it is
more of a challenge for Caperton to read people's names. He frankly says, "I
have a hard time introducing people from China and Japan and using words

that are very different for me." Even with practice that aspect of his job is very challenging.

Jack Horner, who reads to keep up with new information in the field of paleontology, revealed, "I know when I read, I read words. I read one word, then the next word, then the next word. I don't read sentences or paragraphs or books or pages. I read words. It flows better when I read out loud. I can read for quite a ways and then it starts to slow down. . . . I still think reading is the hardest thing I do in my life." Gavin Newsom explained his strategy in reading books. "I'll take a beautiful book and I underline every conceivable page. I read and re-read what I have done. I'm still struggling with dyslexia in multiple ways, and I can't believe I'm still struggling. I can sit there and read a book and not remember two words. I will be daydreaming and still reading. So I force myself to underline like a textbook. It's the only way I can concentrate. What I have to do is re-read it, but when I re-read it, it's captured." Newsom's overall view of his reading is quite positive. "Now I read more than most people . . . people can read faster, but I can read really well. You can mix up all the words and get meaning out of it."

Neil Smith assesses his reading progress over the years. "I kind of outgrew it [but] I don't think it will ever go away because I still don't read at the level of an adult. I still feel I could read at a much higher level, but I tell you I have gotten so much better over the years." Goodkind simply adds, "I wish I could read faster so I could read more things". At times he does misread things. He conveyed very frankly, "I read the title of Dean Koontz's book, on the front of the book, "Counted Shadows" instead of "Counted Sorrows".

Terry Goodkind said about his writing, "I need to work around my dyslexia. One thing I could never do is grammar. I couldn't learn all the rules and diagram sentences. To this day my copy editor calls up and starts using all these words as parts of sentences. I don't know what a participle is. At its root I use grammar through logic to make a sentence more understandable, how to add clarity to the written word. My copy editor now says that I have the cleanest manuscripts she's ever seen."

Spelling is an issue that goes beyond the school-age years as well. Henry Winkler pointed that out, "Spelling is out of the question. For many years I would have to rewrite letters and find different ways of saying things. Because I couldn't figure out how to spell a word. Nor could I find it in the dictionary." Goodkind, who is an admitted poor speller, shared his strategy. "I can't spell so I learned to use the computer to get around the problem." Gavin Newsom also struggles with spelling ". . . and spelling, spelling's just a joke. . . ," he says, "When I see it I know [if] it's spelled right or wrong, but when I write it I can't bloody do it. "

Only one of the extraordinary adults we interviewed told us math is an ongoing challenge. Chuck Close revealed, "I never learned to add, subtract or multiply. It would be a problem like 6 plus 5 which anybody else could do in their head, and I couldn't add those numbers if I had the rest of the day." Several of our interviewees described confusion with numbers and letters. Florence Haseltine relates, "My kids know if I give them a phone number and it's wrong, they'll interchange the last two numbers because that's what I usually do. I don't interchange the middle [numbers], only the last two." Smith tells of a similar experience. "Sometimes I might be writing down a phone number and I'm saying 98, and I'm writing 89." Kendrick Meek has shared how his transposition of numbers and letters provided challenges in his work as a state trooper in Florida. "My words and letters come out backwards from time to time. When I was a state trooper I knew that 65 was the speed limit not 56. I'm able to correct myself." Diane Swonk who deals with numbers every day as an economist speaks of her reversal of statistics. "I'm a dyslexic economist. I don't like to say too many numbers because if the Fed Funds rate is 1.4, 4.0 or .40 you can flip those numbers. I often say my favorite quarter is one where growth is 3.3 per cent because I can't mess up."

Then there are other day-to-day obstacles that spring from having learning disabilities. Close, who admittedly struggles with selective memory, explained his difficulty recognizing faces. "If I were to sit down and have dinner with you I would sit, stare at your face, remember where your children go to school, all kinds of things I will remember forever. But if I see you on the street the next day I would have no memory of ever seeing you before. . . . The memory bank empties out after a certain length of time." This from one of the world's most acclaimed artists, who specializes in painting faces! Swonk speaks of her experience after arriving at the office where she's worked for 19 years. "Every day I get off the elevator and don't know which direction to turn to go to my office. I look for cues to help me compensate."

Henry Winkler tells of his trials and tribulations with driving and organization. "I'm doing a play downtown. In L.A., I'm driving home, and I'm on the wrong freeway. I have to be very organized so I know where everything is. Even in the chaos. But I have to constantly go through my drawers to remember that I have what I have." Similarly, Swonk relates that when she's driving, her kids often jokingly have to tell her to turn to her "other right."

The refreshing thing about the challenges listed above is that they appear to be "small bumps in the road" for the people with learning disabilities in this book. Unlike their childhood experiences, residual issues do not seem to prevent them from doing what they do best, and thankfully so. When they face tasks such as reading or writing, they deal with them, without diminishing their adaptability or productivity. In fact, they seem to expect and accept these glitches, mainly because they can occur every day in a variety of adult settings. Moreover, when learning disabilities or dyslexia do manifest themselves, other adults seem to understand and *they* accommodate to the issue at hand.

Success has its perks. These individuals are so charismatic, so creative, and so extraordinary that they have developed a "track record" that apparently allows for peers, support staff and their families to give them a "pass". To have crossed over to the other side where mistakes are simply mistakes and are not seen as the result of being dumb, lazy, or unmotivated is a very advantageous place to be. The old axiom that success breeds success holds here. This observation has been mentioned in other studies that investigated highly successful individuals with learning disabilities.

It is important to emphasize that despite a high level of success, many of the challenges associated with learning disabilities found in the earlier years do not go away. That phenomenon has been labeled "persisting problems" in Gerber's work that is typically found throughout the life span. Some may simply fade with time, others may be mastered over time, and some may not occur in adult contexts because there is no need to call on them anymore. However, it is unrealistic to assume that the issues found earlier in life no longer affect functioning in later life. The comments by those quoted in this book are testimony to the persistence of dyslexia and other learning disabilities in adulthood.

Chapter 5

RECOLLECTIONS OF BEING A STUDENT

*I would fill a bathtub to the top with hot water, make the room dark and put a
board across the top of the tub, a book rack on the board, and shine a bright
light on the book. I would read every page out loud five times so I could hear
it. I would stay in the bathtub all night long until I was a prune and then hurl
myself out of the water in the morning and run to class.*

— Chuck Close, Photorealist Painter

Their achievements in adulthood are legendary. As children, however,
their experiences in mastering the tasks needed for success in school were
quite challenging, to say the least. Those challenges have much to do with the
nexus of their learning disabilities and the requirements of the K-12
curriculum.

Issues with memorization, drill and repetition, reading, and basic math
highlight their gripping stories of trying to make it in school. Chuck Close told
us about the "sensory deprivation tank" strategy he devised to memorize
material for tests. "I would fill a bathtub to the top with hot water, make the
room dark and put a board across the top of the tub, a book rack on the board,
and shine a bright light on the book. I would read every page out loud five
times so I could hear it. I would stay in the bathtub all night long until I was a
prune and then hurl myself out of the water in the morning and run to class. I
might possibly be able to remember to get through the exam. If the test was
postponed for a week, I would have to repeat the same process."

Kendrick Meek remembers having trouble learning basic facts. "If you
haven't had the repetition, you have not had the opportunity of introducing
new things. You start knowing mathematical problems, you start knowing five
times five is twenty-five, or five times six is thirty, versus your numbers

getting turned around. You are putting zero, three or something. You could easily get it wrong. I didn't use the right mathematical equation to do forty-six rather than a sixty-four. But you know one can get confused".

Learning to read, and reading to learn, proved to be two of the most challenging issues of their school years. Jack Horner describes how it affected him. "I don't know if anyone realized I could not read. They knew something was wrong, but I don't think I gave away that I could not actually read. I wouldn't read out loud because I couldn't. You can get a lot of information even if you can't read, especially the way the school system works. . . . Everybody kept saying why don't you take wood or metal shop or something simple, but that's not what I was interested in. I was really interested in science even though I knew I wouldn't get a good grade."

Terry Goodkind also described his experiences of reading while in school. "I had difficulty in reading and that made school difficult. The teachers said that I wasn't trying hard enough. I could understand if I could read at my own pace. The teachers didn't understand that. Their approach was: You have thirty seconds to read this passage and answer the questions. I couldn't understand the paragraph in thirty seconds." Goodkind also recalls how the joy was taken out of reading for him. "I remember the 'Lady in the Lake' poem by Byron. I read it and thought how cool the story was. Then they started dissecting it word by word, sentence by sentence. They made something beautiful into a mush of technical things. They expected you to learn, and they destroyed the value of what I thought the written word was. I was very frustrated with that kind of thing. To me reading was torture, it was boring, it was diagramming sentences. It was taking life out of the piece, and it was a horrible experience." Charles Schwab spoke about his love for reading by accessing a different kind of reading material. "What I really loved in my early childhood was reading classic comic books. I lived off those because I was an incredibly slow reader. So the early part of my reading, my best reading, was using classic comic books. I would go over and over them again, the same classic comic books." This approach also provided support when he read the conventional books used for instruction.

One of the most inventive reading strategies comes from Patricia Polacco, the illustrator and story-teller. Her strategy for reading resulted from her interactions with her favorite teacher, George Falker, in seventh grade. "What you perceive is different than what other people see. I get to a point where you ask me how I read, I read by looking at the negative space around the words. George Falker put me in front of the words of M.C. Escher. That helped me more than the Orton-Gillingham method [a remedial reading intervention for dyslexics] or anything else you can imagine. I understood that you can have more positive and negative space, and the words weren't shaped that way. They were going in and out of my field of vision. So when I stop, I am still looking at the pattern around the word."

It is not surprising that those we interviewed shared few positive memories from their school-age years. In fact, the challenges of reading and "keeping up" were chronic issues that led to doubts and low self-esteem about their academic potential. The people we have written about had brilliance within them, but rarely had an opportunity to show it, seldom receiving accolades for their achievements. Consistent performance was typically not part of their school experience, and low expectations seemed to drive the educational approach devised for them. This is highlighted by the suggestions teachers made to Chuck Close and Jack Horner (during middle school) that vocational education seemed to be their only possible path to a productive life. One wonders what Jack Horner was thinking while he was failing science and winning annual science fairs.

How wonderful it was for some of them to be rescued by teachers who understood them and their struggles! Interestingly, it is Terry Goodkind and Patricia Polacco who were very much inspired by the English teachers who helped them see beyond their basic issues with reading and language. It is ironic that they both are noted writers in their own right and currently at the top of their game.

The comments of the 12 highly successful individuals we interviewed remind us of research findings in several other studies about adults with learning disabilities. It appears that for the most part, those we interviewed did not see the value in their early education. They simply felt that there was a disconnect between what they learned in school and what they found to be valuable in their years after leaving school. This leads one to believe that perhaps K-12 education really did not contribute to their ultimate success. Not surprisingly, those who succeeded in college and graduate/professional programs found value in that part of their education. After all, they had more choices and were able to tailor their programs (and academic majors) to their interests. In fact, no one we interviewed spoke negatively about their higher education experiences. Even Jack Horner, who later received an honorary doctorate in paleontology and is subsequently addressed as doctor or professor (out of deep respect) did not put the blame on the University of Montana for his very poor undergraduate performance. In fact he has the highest regard for the chair of the university's geology department.

There is no substitute for confidence in fostering achievement and success. Moreover, it has a significant impact on motivation. That confidence, however, was absent earlier in their educational experience. It seems that success fueled success, but that did not come to fruition until adulthood. In fact, in the case of the writers mentioned above, it did not come until their mid-forties. Sometimes it takes a while to be successful. The key seems to be having "something in the tank" when leaving high school so that one can continue on without feeling defeated or being driven by the insidious dynamic of learned helplessness (feeling anything that is done will not have value or a positive result). Perhaps we can say these accomplished people are not only prototypes for success but they are also survivors.

Chapter 6

NOW AND THEN

It took me a long time to think that I was smart.
— Gaston Caperton, Politician, Educational Leader

I felt so different. I spent so much of my childhood hiding my secret.
In adulthood I realized my strengths and went 180 degrees from hiding it,
to wearing it on my shoulder.
— Diane Swonk, Business Economist

The differences between childhood and adulthood are profound. When learning disabilities enter into the equation, these differences appear to be even more profound. In childhood and adolescence, the focus on attaining educational goals and developing skills become the foundation of adjustment for the adult years. Adulthood, on the other hand, is more complex and not as easily characterized. The givens, however, are more autonomy, more choices, and myriad interwoven issues, which combine to make up the adult experience.

The adults we interviewed saw their school- and beyond school-years as dramatically different. When asked about the difference between his childhood and adulthood Chuck Close put it succinctly. He simply said, "Everything, everything, everything!" The overriding message of several who were interviewed was the confidence they found in adulthood, particularly with their extraordinary success. Gavin Newsom commented that he had very little confidence as a child, whereas in adulthood he found confidence that was a great source of strength for him. He realized his "strengths and capacities and their benefits". Patricia Polacco framed her thoughts in a more provocative manner. "I'm fearless now, whereas before I was timid. Now I don't care what people think". Charles Schwab remarked that he could deal with his dyslexia more confidently in adulthood which, he added, "is a very comforting thing for me". It was Henry Winkler who described his lack of confidence in childhood with an interesting twist. He observed, "It took a long time for me to gain confidence." He then proceeded to explain that his character of "The Fonz" in the popular television show *Happy Days* was his alter ego. It was so easy for him to craft the role of the super cool and confident Fonz since he had been the polar opposite during his younger years.

For others adulthood provided clarity about the manifestations of their learning disabilities. Neil Smith readily shared that during childhood he "didn't know what was wrong, which was very confusing". Only as an adult did he gain clarity about the challenges of his dyslexia. Terry Goodkind described a childhood in which he was frustrated with learning, particularly his inability to read fast enough. That issue tended to subside during his adult years. In each of their comments there was an undertone of questioning their intelligence. Gaston Caperton summed it up well saying, "It took me a long time to think that I was smart". In his adult years as he became more and more successful he viewed his dyslexia only as an inconvenience. Failure was the self-attribution Florence Haseltine held onto during her childhood. In part, this notion was reinforced by her mother as well as her peers as she was "one who did not fit in". As she became more and more successful in her medical training and subsequently her career that feeling began to subside.

All these extraordinary adults with learning disabilities felt they were "different", which led some to feel ashamed. As a result, much of their childhood experience was one of trying to hide something uncomfortable while at the same time striving to be a "regular kid". It was only in adulthood that accomplishment and success reversed that feeling. As Diane Swonk put it so well, "I felt so different. I spent so much of my childhood hiding my secret. In adulthood I realized my strengths and went 180 degrees from hiding it, to wearing it on my shoulder".

Childhood can be a very confusing time, particularly if dyslexia and other learning disabilities are part of that experience. So much is predicated on school achievement that one's childhood can become very complicated to figure out. Learning disabilities can also overshadow other important aspects of the childhood. Learning disabilities can be like a game of "whack-a mole"; when one issue is dealt with, another is just around the corner. And that can happen day after day, for years on end.

There is something notable about adulthood for the people in this book which coincides with findings from other studies about success and learning disabilities. As adults, these individuals appear to have a greater capacity for self-awareness and introspective thought. Those who become successful understand how their learning disability factored into their lives. They seem to know full well what their challenges are and how to compensate for them. If they cannot compensate, they know how and where to get help. Fortunately for many of them, they have assistants who are important in supporting their activities. That support allows them to be more effective and efficient in their work. Therefore, it seems they are not thrown by their challenges, but are readily able to deal with them.

Most important, with their success and celebrity, they are at ease with their challenges because learning disabilities have become only a part of their lives, but not the larger part of who they are. They can remind themselves that they have learning disabilities while also being a MacArthur Fellowship winner, a Super Bowl Champion, a Golden Globe winner or a well-known name in investing and philanthropy.

Perhaps the most significant difference between childhood and adulthood is having more control of one's life. We can make the choices that suit us, both professionally and personally. For the individuals we interviewed, success gives them even more control than the average adult, but that is the reward of the work they have done and the success they have achieved. Their passions and their energies can be directed to where they think they are most fruitful. One success leads to another. How different from their childhood experience. The "best of times and worst of times" (as Charles Dickens put it) is an apt description of adults with learning disabilities. Such is the experience of those who are extraordinarily successful despite their challenges.

Chapter 7

FINDING A NICHE

I didn't figure out what I do best, I just did the thing I loved best.
— Professor Jack Horner, Paleontologist

Becoming successful is a process that begins far earlier than one's first adult achievements. In many ways success depends on making the right choices in deciding how strengths are parlayed into an area in which one has interest, skills, motivation, and passion and (sometimes) experience. It is safe to say that the adults who have achieved extraordinary levels of success have found their niches, another way of describing "goodness of fit". It is with this "fit" that one reaches the realization of what can be done and what is possible. Finding one's niche involves making a conscious effort to stay away from areas that are too challenging and in which there is little likelihood of developing sufficient skills. It is a matter of avoiding areas and situations/environments that emphasize or accentuate one's difficulties/ deficits. At the same time it requires choosing areas and contexts that play to, and capitalize on, their strengths and special talents. All the research and writing in the area of success and adults with learning disabilities emphasizes that finding the right niche is key in finding success.

However, such choices are not always clear and obvious. Caution should be taken in assuming that having "weak skills" in certain areas should preclude someone from specific career choices. What if Terry Goodkind and Patricia Polacco chose not to be writers because of their dyslexia? Or Chuck Close not to paint portraits because he had a poor memory for faces? It would certainly have interfered with their abilities to live satisfying and rewarding lives. And what a loss this would have been for the rest of us. Well-meaning teachers and counselors who steer students away from specific pursuits because they may struggle should heed this note of caution.

Some of the successful people we interviewed discovered their niches early in childhood. From his earliest memories Henry Winkler wanted to be an actor. He related," I knew when I was young, lying in bed, in New York City, before I fell asleep. I dreamt, I ate, I slept, I brushed my teeth, with this dream of being an actor. It was bigger than I was. Sometimes it was so intense." Those sentiments are similar to those voiced by Jack Horner whose earliest memories are of playing in his father's gravel pit in Montana, "I didn't figure out what I do best, I just did the thing I loved best. I wanted to be a paleontologist for as long as I can remember. I think I was born this way. There was no 'Plan B' ever. . . . Even if I sat on an oil well I would consider myself a paleontologist, even if I was driving a truck. If I had a big 18-wheeler and I was driving around I would still consider myself a paleontologist."

Chuck Close shared an early memory of his father taking him to Sears to buy his first paint set. He always enjoyed art and used it in grade school to create projects that helped him earn passing grades. His talent became even more apparent when he attended the University of Washington as an undergraduate. "I was screwed in things like marine biology. I couldn't remember the phylum, genus and species. All these things looked alike. I dropped biology, I dropped marine biology, all those things because I couldn't . . . I found geology which was more visual, better because you could see the earth unfolding. It was very visual to me and that I could do. I dropped a lot of courses when I found it wasn't going to work. God knows how I made it through school." It was apparent what his niche was, however. "Then I got scholarships and won prizes and actually graduated the University of Washington with the highest grade point average in the School of Art. I couldn't believe." As noted previously, he went on to continue his studies at Yale University School of Design.

By contrast, some of the successful adults we met didn't discover their niches until later adulthood. Such is the case for the two writers Terry Goodkind and Patricia Polacco. Goodkind, who began writing at age 45, says that while in school he always wanted to be a writer. However, school did nothing to help him pursue that dream. "When I was in school I didn't write things down because teachers would criticize what I wrote because my spelling and grammar were so bad. I had such trouble reading that I just didn't want to go there because it was inviting criticism. But I loved stories and making up stories. I'd tell them to myself in my head. There were all these stories in my head. . . . I always wanted to be a writer. I thought writing novels was the most noble thing I could do." Polacco related that many of her stories came from her experience growing up in a colorful family of storytellers. She started writing books as an adult, when her writing skill began to match her extraordinary ability as an illustrator. She readily admits she found her niche "by doing it. I loved writing and illustrating". Her success was fueled by writing to motivate children who shared similar school experiences. "There was a book store in San Jose that started sending me out to talk to schools, and I realized how many children there are like me and there was nobody speaking for them. There was nobody to tell them that they were going to be all right. That was finding my niche . . . . They need to see someone successful who had a hard time in school . . . I would say that's how it all began at about the age of 43 or 44."

Our own research has shown that self-awareness is a key ingredient in finding one's niche, and finding one's niche is related to life success. Gaston Caperton's thinking illustrates this. "A niche," he says, "is what comes naturally. . . If I tried to be an accountant, I do not think I would have been a good accountant. I started out in the insurance business and found out I was a good communicator, that I am a good salesperson. I know how to get along with people. I knew I was a good athlete and people followed me, that I could inspire people. You kind of build on your own successes. You follow your strengths. Don't try to do something you're not." This kind of introspective thinking led him to eventually become a leader as the governor of West Virginia.

It is also important to point out that finding one's niche can be serendipitous – something that isn't planned. The challenge in finding one's niche via this route is recognizing it when it happens. Diane Swonk makes the point of saying that she found her niche by accident when she enrolled in her first economics class as an undergraduate. "By taking economics by accident, I found it gave a sort of clarity to this chaos I had grown up in. I realized I didn't have to be the way it was if better economic policies had been in place. It was so natural." She also shared the genesis of her interest in economics. "My mom was an artist and my dad was a strategist and an engineer. Economics was sort of a creative application of math . . . . My parents were so involved in current events, so it was the epitome of everything I grew up with." Economics is a field that is broad in theory and application. When asked if she chose the "niche within the niche" she explained, "I'm not suited to accounting. It's very micro, very detail-oriented, not big world, big picture. My background is in labor economics which is micro. But it is the study of workers in the workplace and how they react to management. Even though it's kind of micro, it's also macro."

Charles Schwab specifically uses the word "serendipity" to explain how he found his niche. "I think the serendipity of it all probably came from reading the biographies of famous people. I knew I wanted to be successful in life, and the measurement was making money. My father was a lawyer but my parents talked about how things were tight because we were coming out of a Depression. It was the war years. So I put two and two together and said I don't want to be like that. I wanted to have enough money. So how do people make money? I sort of went down that path. So for by whatever sense of luck I fell into the investment area."

The classic question, "What do you want to be when you grow up?" is difficult for anyone to answer. Even today, with such dire national economic conditions, qualified people cannot find work in their areas of expertise. Ultimately, a career path can be a surprise to all, including oneself. So it is wise to think about the concept of finding a niche in the same way. The process of finding one's niche takes time. It is a process of sorting out interests, abilities, talents, strengths and weaknesses. It is also tied to personal motivation and modeling from others in one's life. Luck and serendipity also become part of the mix from time to time.

So we should not be surprised that Jack Horner found his niche in his "own backyard" via his experience in the gravel pits of Montana, a place where eons earlier dinosaurs flourished. Then there is the case of Chuck Close who showed artistic talent from the age of seven, received his first easel from his father, and developed his artistic skills and style over a lifetime. While Florence Haseltine was a gifted student in math and science, the challenges of reading and language diminished her overall academic profile. Yet she persevered and parlayed her strengths into a distinguished medical career. Of course, size, strength and speed can lead one into a niche that has a trajectory to the NFL. Neil Smith's story provides an excellent example of that career path, yet his role as football executive came as a surprise. After all, how many former NFL players continue on as executives? The most common route is to become a sports announcer or analyst. Even as a teenager, Henry Winkler wanted to be an actor. So did many other would-be actors who never "made it". But how can one go from American icon to director/producer and writer? Certainly, his skill set for roles behind the camera were honed while he spent many successful years in front of the camera, as the star of the number one rated T.V. show of its time.

Gaston Caperton, Gavin Newsom, and Charles Schwab found their niches over time. Entrepreneurs see opportunities that can be parlayed into successful endeavors. When Gavin Newsom was a successful wine merchant in San Francisco, did he really have his eye on the becoming mayor? Similarly when Gaston Caperton began selling insurance in West Virginia did he really think it would lead to the governorship of his state or becoming the president of the prestigious College Board?

Then there is the aforementioned adult fiction writer Terry Goodkind and children's author and illustrator Patricia Polacco. There is something to be said to becoming what you hoped you would become, no matter when it happens. Both followed other interests before they found their "true" niches. Prior to her success, Polacco received a Ph.D. in art history, while Goodkind was a painter (fine arts) and even built his own house.

Finding one's niche can be likened to finding one's life partner. It is a match that has both objective and subjective criteria. It is dynamic and unpredictable. There is no blueprint, nor is there a guarantee of success. Clearly, the people chronicled in this book were destined for success because of their intellect, resourcefulness, special talents, and drive. Their examples are a testament to finding their niches and making the most of many possibilities.

It is interesting to note that each of the people in this book appear to be both passionate about what they do and to have a special talent. However, it is possible to be talented in an area without having a passion for pursuing it. Conversely, one may not have a special ability in a certain area yet be passionate about what they do. The extent that the absence of one characteristic, either talent or passion, might counteract the other and help lead people with learning difficulties to the road to success cannot be determined by our interviews. Moreover, is it not the intention of this book to make such a determination. Such an interesting notion will require further investigation.

Chapter 8

CAN DYSLEXIA AND OTHER LEARNING DISABILITIES BE CONSIDERED A GIFT?

It is a gift alright, but it is a horrifying gift. If one side of my brain is shutting down, the artistic part accelerates. I can see and understand things that other people can't. It sounds egotistical, but it is genius to be able to evaluate and understand things that maybe other people aren't getting.
— Patricia Polacco, Children's Author and Illustrator

It seems paradoxical to combine the concepts of "gift" and "learning disabilities." Can they really exist simultaneously? How can they be related? From one perspective, having learning problem drives an individual to function and behave in certain ways. In other words, a learning disability might lead to particular abilities, sensitivities, or skills. People with disabilities sometimes develop extraordinary talents and skills because they are denied certain cognitive, sensory or physical functions. For example, there are stories of people who lose their vision but develop a keen sense of hearing as a way to compensate. Even cases of autistic savants lead some to think that what is lost in one area may be more than gained in another through extraordinary talents or skills (such as math, memory, art, music). Above and beyond special talents, this view also lends itself to the idea that the struggles inherent in dealing with a learning disability might promote increased empathy and compassion for others, or foster a "fighting spirit" from having to face and push through hardship.

Another perspective proposes that the same neurobiological differences that may be responsible for the difficulties experienced by persons with learning problems might also be responsible for the extraordinary talents and abilities which are often seen in these individuals. Interviewees cited special talents including highly developed visual thinking, visual spatial abilities, as well as the ability to "think out of the box" or "see the big picture." In this view, such talents are thought of as being innate or inherent in the individual. Still another view of the relationship between learning disabilities and special talents contends that the exceptional talents shown by some individuals with learning disabilities are merely coincidental and that the two "conditions" just happen to independently co-exist as they may in any person without a disability.

Some studies suggest that people with learning disabilities, dyslexia specifically, have exceptional gifts or talents that are not necessarily found in the general population.[1] However, there is no body of evidence that clearly proves or disproves such theories. It is not our intention to comment or conjecture regarding the relative merits of these theories or the limited research that currently exists. Rather, our aim is to share the insiders' perspectives —in their own words— regarding the relationship between simultaneously having a gift or talent and a learning difficulty.

These extraordinary individuals responded to the question of "whether learning disabilities/dyslexia can be considered a gift" in two ways. First, that the presence and the experience of living with learning difficulties results in positive characteristics, traits, behaviors, or "lessons learned" that may not have occurred if they did not have it. Second, that there was "another side of the coin" in having learning disabilities/dyslexia, that is, that some special talents or abilities appear to be an integral part of their learning difficulties. Both scenarios are possible. Although Chuck Close does not think of his learning issues as a gift, at the same time he exclaimed, "I don't think it was a disaster." He went on to say, "Would I have liked it easier? It' s f---ing hard getting through life not knowing who you are talking to, never remembering where you are going, not remembering a name. I think it is a little disingenuous when people say that it is the best thing that ever happened to them. But there is a gift in this. It changes the way you deal with life". This adaptive aspect was echoed by Florence Haseltine. "Bull ---- ! But it allows you to adapt quickly to difficult situations. . . . I always know there is more than one way to do anything." Charles Schwab also cast aside the idea of a gift when he described his struggles while in school. "I sure did not think of it as a

---

[1] Geiger, G. & Lettvin, J. Y. (1987). Peripheral vision in persons with dyslexia. *New England Journal of Medicine*, 316, 1238-1243.

von Karolyi, C., Winner, E. Gray, W., & Sherman, G. F. (2003). Dyslexia linked to talent: Global visual-spatial ability. *Brain and Language*, 85, 427-431.

gift. I thought it was a major handicap when I went to college and I couldn't keep up with the reading and writing. It was all I could do to stay alive in school". Gaston Caperton viewed the idea of a gift from multiple perspectives. "You don't think of it as a gift. But I think the challenges in life and the ability to overcome adversity is a critically important part of anybody's success. For example, Franklin Roosevelt they said was not a great man until he was crippled. Overcoming and dealing with that made him a much more compassionate and determined person. I don't think of it as an asset when I get up to give a speech and can't read. Or I don't think of it as an asset when I am with other people whose brain is different than mine and can remember everything they read, memorize much easier than I do. They have a much more brilliant mind than I do."

Some statements did reflect that a learning disability might be a gift. Henry Winkler simply said, "That's probably true . . . for the longest time, I wanted to carve it out of my brain . . . scoop it out with a spoon, like a damaged part. But it finally dawned on me that maybe I wouldn't have been able to achieve [what I have] without the force of having to fight my learning challenge." Both Kendrick Meek and Gavin Newsom believe that it made them different from others in a positive way. Meek shared that the gift of his learning disability allowed him "to think differently than everyone else, a different mindset." Newsom exclaimed, "When I think about a gift, God, I am so blessed to have these struggles because if I didn't I think I would be average in doing everything or lots of things. I have found I have a little more aptitude than most in some other things, which is marvelous."

Others definitely saw their learning disabilities as a gift and credited having a disability as helping them discover what they can do. Patricia Polacco related, "I would say it is a gift alright, but it is a horrifying gift. . . . if one side of my brain is shutting down, the other part accelerates and goes into hyper-drive. That then accelerates the . . . artistic side. . . . There are things I can do visually. I can see and understand things that other people can't. And I realize, please understand how I am saying this, is a type of genius. Sounds egotistical, but it is genius to be able to evaluate and understand things that maybe other people aren't getting."

Diane Swonk sees her learning disability as a gift in the way she approaches her work as an economist. "There is no question that it is a gift. It has evolved in my life from a hindrance to a gift. It's the way that I think about the world, and I get paid to think about the world the way I do. For many people the reason they cannot do what I do is because they think in a line. She went on to explain, "I think multi-dimensionally, and I have learned that is a dyslexic trait. I do not think linearly. In economics it's like a butterfly one place can create a hurricane somewhere else. That's how my mind works, and I am well suited to what I do because I think in a multi-dimensional, interactive, simultaneous equation. Not everybody can do that and so thank goodness I can do that". Like others in this study, Gavin Newsom mentions that he is able to think "three-dimensionally and can often visualize something before it actually appears." Florence Haseltine speaks of her ability to "get the big picture" when making a decision and not get bogged down by a lot of detail. She also contends that she doesn't "think out of the box" as some people might describe it, but more "bouncing around the box." In contrast, Chuck Close, who is considered to be a genius in the visual arts speaks of how he has difficulty recognizing faces in three dimensions, how he needs to make portraits flat and to break things down into small parts because he is overwhelmed by the "whole."

Jack Horner attributes his approach as a research paleontologist to the gift within his dyslexia. "I agree one hundred per cent. Here is a good example: There are a lot of books here [in his research office]. But that is other people's information, other people's ideas. So most non-dyslexic people would read all this crap and would have in their head everybody else's ideas and not their own. A dyslexic is not going to read all this crap .They are going to read little bits and pieces and do a lot of figuring on their own and then come up with some really cool ideas that no one else has. I think dyslexics are good at synthesizing. Taking pieces from here and there and adding them all together. And I would claim that a genius is a dyslexic and a non-dyslexic together, the synthesis is the creative side. So that is what I call genius. I don't think you have genius without a dyslexic side". It is Terry Goodkind who directly links the gift of his dyslexia to the success of his writing style. "I think my books connect with people because I had trouble reading. I understanding what kept me from not reading. And I wrote books from a dyslexic's perceptive. Because when I am writing for an audience, I am writing for myself. I am telling myself a story. So I am telling the story to a dyslexic."

The concept of a gift can have multiple meanings. No doubt all the perspectives above represent the thinking of individuals who have successfully reframed their learning disability in a positive way. In the words of Chuck Close, they "celebrate their strengths" rather than focusing on their challenges. Without question the struggle of overcoming a learning disability has the potential to make one stronger and provide self-confidence. That is revealed in the thoughts above. These extraordinary adults also expressed that learning disabilities have given them a way of thinking that facilitates their achievements. Some say it is "thinking out of the box". The question is: Does this kind of thinking come naturally from a mind that conceptualizes the world differently because of what is called a learning "disability"?

Clearly not all of the individuals in our study believe that a learning disability/dyslexia actually is a gift. Some are vehemently opposed to the notion that their learning disabilities were a gift and cited the hardships and struggles they faced as a result of having to cope with it. Others clearly expressed that it was a gift and were thankful for its presence. Furthermore, several of these extraordinary people believed that they did possess inherent differences from people without learning issues– possibly a "different side of the same dyslexia coin" that resulted in special visual and artistic talents. It is important to keep in mind that there is no single view expressed by these individuals regarding learning disabilities as a gift; one size does not fit all. At the same time, there is little doubt that, for each of these individuals, their learning difficulties served to shape who they are– their behaviors, choices, personalities, life philosophies, world views and perhaps special gifts.

Chapter 9

PROBLEM-SOLVING AS A WAY OF LIFE

I don't dwell on problems, I deal with problems. . . .The fact that [my] learning disability did not get in my way gave me a belief I could overcome problems.

– Gaston Caperton, Politician, Educational Leader

One of the most traumatic events in my life was surviving the World Trade Center [collapse]. I've been lost a lot being a dyslexic . . . but I ran from the World Trade Center and got twenty people out with me. People were sort of amazed at my willingness to . . . take charge and grab everyone to follow me.

– Diane Swonk, Business Economist

In Gerber's prior studies on highly successful adults with learning disabilities one of several ingredients found in their profiles was learned creativity. In essence, creativity emerged as one of the main assets that allowed for greater achievement in adulthood when compared to peers without learning difficulties. Learned creativity is characterized as something that develops over time, stemming from the "learning disabled experience". The process of problem-solving evolves through navigating the daily challenges that people with learning disabilities encounter each day. Some highly successful adults believe it is something in them that, figuratively speaking, "tries to build a better mousetrap." Patricia Polacco identifies significant problem-solving abilities as a gift; this idea is borne out by some of the other extraordinary adults we interviewed for this book. Whether this can be considered a gift found in the complexities of learning disabilities is debatable.

Effective problem-solving can be seen in the work of Gaston Caperton when he was governor as well as CEO of the College Board. "I think I am a good visionary. I can see the future well. . . . I have good intuition and a lot of it came from being dyslexic." He goes on to say, "I don't spend much of my life thinking about things as being problems. . . . I don't *dwell* on problems, I *deal* with problems. I think you are able to overcome something that was difficult when you deal with the problem. And you can deal with them successfully." He continues, "The fact that I had a learning disability did not get in my way and gave me a belief I could overcome problems. I wasn't scared of problems."

Chuck Close viewed his problem-solving abilities as being part of his own creative process. "I was maybe more interesting ultimately because of my learning disabilities. It made my work different from [that of] other people. Once you know what art looks like it's not hard to make some of it. It's gonna look like someone else's art. If you are a problem creator and not only a problem solver, if you ask yourself interesting questions that no one else answers, then you are out there by yourself. People see you as being unique, idiosyncratic and whatever. Everyone's trying to solve the same problems with the same solutions. My solutions never fit. So I figured, why should I try to solve someone else's problems? I'll go make my own problems." That seemed to be true for Jack Horner as well in his work as a ground-breaking paleontologist. "It's easy to tell when a person has read somebody else's stuff. They don't have original thoughts themselves. So I think I am pretty good at figuring out things. But I am slow. It takes me a while to figure things out. . . . I find problems more fun than anything. When people say I can't do something, that's a challenge and it is fun figuring it out." Diane Swonk describes her problem-solving abilities in terms of being an economist. "Being a problem solver is so important to what is happening in the economy today." Her thinking is as unique as her problem-solving abilities. "I'll never forget the quote in the *Forbes* ["Dyslexic CEO"] article. Chuck Schwab said 'I always know the ending, and I had to walk everyone else in the room through it.' That's exactly right. I am constantly figuring out the end game".

Part of Swonk's thinking also hints of problem-solving abilities to work around difficulties. "You have to overcome obstacles. That in itself makes you a leader. The important thing to understand is that it is your challenge and your ability to overcome them. That is what makes you a problem solver." Goodkind related that he finds a way around problems simply by finding a solution to them. A famous saying in one of his books stems straight from that philosophy. The wizard says to his grandson, "Think of the solution, not of the problem." According to Goodkind people are often too focused on the problem, and thinks that dyslexia is framed that way. Ultimately, the problem-solving in Goodkind's opinion is very pragmatic - "just working around the problem to get things done."

Problem-solving also seems to be a source of motivation for not "failing". Patricia Polacco's words show how determination can be the lifeblood of achievement. "I am bound and determined. I am going to do it and I'll figure out a way. . . . Problem-solving. I can look at things and understand because of my understanding of congruency. If I visualize it and I believe it, trust me, it's going to happen, hell or high water."

An amazing problem-solving example was conveyed by Diane Swonk involving the tragic day of September 11th, 2001. "One of the most traumatic events in my life was surviving the [attack on the] World Trade Center. I've been lost a lot being a dyslexic. I'm always lost and finding my way out. My dad used to teach me tricks to figure how to get where I really needed to go even though I was lost. So being lost doesn't scare me. Running from the World Trade Center and getting twenty people out with me. People were sort of amazed at my willingness to just sort of take charge and grab everyone to follow me. . . . Dyslexia played a role in it because I was so comfortable not knowing where I was going and just going there anyway and getting away from danger. So, that part I think was a role of having my whole life plowing ahead no matter what. We all fail in life, part of it is picking yourself up and dusting yourself off and keep going".

As previously mentioned, prior research indicates that, for adults with learning difficulties, learned creativity is a key ingredient in attaining success, and at its core are significant problem-solving abilities. It was present in all who Gerber studied and was seen to a smaller degree in those persons who were less successful in their adult lives. The other side of the continuum was learned helplessness characterized by a mindset of defeat, a sense of being powerless, and a reluctance to take on new challenges. In essence, a big part of being a successful adult with learning disabilities is an almost constant engagement in thinking differently. The question is which came first, thinking differently because of unconventional cognitive abilities (associated with learning disabilities) or highly-developed problem-solving skills because of the need to figure out how to adjust to circumstances and situations that don't fit a more "typical" cognitive style. This weighty question cannot be answered in this book and needs to be answered by further research.

An analysis of our interviews shows individuals who are very creative thinkers. It seems that problem-solving may be one source of their creativity. Jack Horner has revolutionized thinking about evolution with his unique take on dinosaurs nurturing their young. His continued work with dinosaur DNA makes *Jurassic Park* seem not too far from reality. Chuck Close has become one of America's greatest artists because of his problem-solving approach to style and technique stemming from both his specific learning disability and his physical disability. Charles Schwab became a pioneer in retail investing as a result of pragmatic problem-solving for "smaller scale investors" who wanted to participate in the stock market. Diane Swonk uses her problem-solving abilities each day as she converts economic data into meaningful information that has practical relevance for a science that is often noted for being too esoteric.

When interviewing the people in this study we often found ourselves enthralled with the content of their comments and the energy they brought to the conversation. Their responses to the questions were quite unique. We could only come to the conclusion that they had extraordinary successes as a result of seeing the world in a different way; this allowed them to have a "different take" when they engaged in the problem-solving process. They seem to "think outside of the box" as a way of conducting their professional as well as their personal lives. This makes them not only current day exemplars, but visionaries in a world that becomes more complicated every day. Such complexity seems to be a welcome challenge for them while other people may be thrown by it.

Chapter 10

CRITICAL INCIDENTS ALONG THE WAY

My first level of confidence came in my first year of business school. We were doing case studies and . . . had to write an analysis and solution to the problem. I wrote a page and a half, which was long for me. It was the first paper of my first year. Out of two hundred in the class they picked my paper. It gave me this profound feeling. I wasn't as dumb as I thought I was.
— Charles Schwab, Financier and Philanthropist

Prior research on eminent American scientists with disabilities and highly successful adults with learning disabilities has shown that critical incidents have an impact on success. Critical incidents are events that influence, sometimes in profound ways, thoughts about self, choices to be considered, and life paths to be taken. Folded into this somewhat "magical experience" are meanings, both positive and negative, which shape thought and action. Critical incidents can happen at any time during development and can occur many times and in a variety of settings.

Not surprisingly, the critical incidents described by the extraordinary adults in this book have had significant effects on their lives. These critical events often occurred during the school-age years. For example, teachers became the source of motivation, inspiration and understanding. Henry Winkler told us about a high school music teacher who cast him in the Gershwin musical "Of Thee I Sing" because he had "faith in him." It was the first time he participated in an extracurricular activity since his grades were so low. This critical incident was the beginning of a stellar acting career.

Terry Goodkind tells of a teacher who he described as a pivotal person. She took a very different approach in teaching him English, saying, "I don't care how long it takes you to read, I just want you to think about it." He described how he would go to her class and be given things to read that were not for the regular class. "She helped me understand that I could accomplish those kinds of things." Children's author Patricia Polacco wrote one of her most famous books *Thank You Mr. Falker* as a result of a critical incident when she was 14 and in seventh grade. It was Mr. Falker who made her understand her learning disability and all its challenges. She related, "Mr. Falker walked into my life and helped me realize what was going on. . . . I had something with a name, that there were other people like me and that it was not synonymous with being stupid."

Chuck Close described a combination of school-age critical incidents that were a mixture of pain and pleasure. "I couldn't run and I would have sadistic gym teachers that would make me run. I remember [in order] to graduate I had to climb a rope. I couldn't get off the ground, I couldn't. In English I was supposed to memorize a poem. I had the entire year to do it and I could not do it. I was humiliated and asked over and over [to recite it] in public in class. I couldn't do it. So all these imprints that you have about performance, about fitting in, about doing it the way everybody else does it are negatively charged. I ran from the things I couldn't do and celebrated the things I could do. It made everything that I could do more pleasurable [and] so much more important."

Others told us about critical incidents that occurred during college or in advanced professional training. Charles Schwab, after having a very challenging time in his K-12 school years, experienced success in his university experience that framed the years to come. "I guess the first level of confidence came in my first year of business school. We were doing case studies, and I thought and thought about a particular case study. And we had to write an analysis and solution to the problem. I wrote a page and a half, which was long for me. I submitted it. It was the first paper of my first year. Out of two hundred in the class they picked my paper. It gave me this profound feeling. I wasn't as dumb as I thought I was". Another example was shared by Dr. Haseltine who chose her medical specialty as a result of a critical experience. "I think it was when I went into a surgical specialty and not a clinical specialty, like internal medicine. You had to one-up each other in how much you knew and where you read it. I thought it was a theme of one-upmanship that I could never play. . . . If you are a surgeon that doesn't play that kind of role, I could get big fibroids with a two inch incision. I could play that game. So quickly I looked around and decided I was not going into clinical medicine. . . . I picked surgery because you know the effects of surgery right away, not 10 years later. I chose things you could see and feel more than you can feel in intellectual one-upmanship".

For some, the critical incidents they identified did not occur until they had finished their formal education and were into their careers. Neil Smith, who had completed his career in the NFL, said, "I never thought I would be an owner [of a football team]. To get a franchise here [Kansas City] was like a no-brainer for me because it was easy. It was almost like a turning point for me." Kendrick Meek spoke of the realities of employment for persons with learning disabilities. "The first test I took [in the police academy] was on radar. It is not as simple as pressing a button to get a speed reading, it has a lot to do with mathematics, understanding the device, very technical. You could fail two tests in the highway patrol and then you are out. I failed the first test. So I went to the captain who runs the academy and gave him, you know, to talk about Kendrick Meek and learning disabilities and dyslexia. He just boldly looked at me and said, I love you and I think you are going to make a good trooper, but if you fail another test you are out of the academy. It was the reality of the fact, the real world and not an educational setting where people spend a lot of time with you. And the first time it really hit me. I had to do more than the next person. I didn't fail another test!"

Whereas past research on critical incidents hinged on one event or a series of scattered events, a number of the people in this book added a new dimension to the thinking about the impact of critical incidents on adults with learning disabilities. Gaston Caperton explained critical events as more of an "evolutionary thing" as his successes over time gave him the belief that he could overcome problems and not be afraid of them. Patricia Polacco expressed the idea that "every day is fraught with critical incidents when you have a learning disability. Let me tell you, you are always up against something that's a challenge and new. . . . It is not something that once it's over, it's over . . . it's there, it is a struggle."

Jack Horner saw critical incidents as largely irrelevant to his experience. He responded, "I started out one day doing what I wanted to do and have been doing it my whole life. I have been making wonderful discoveries. There is no real point I can say I was successful except when I was 38 years old and *Esquire* magazine picked me as one of the top 200 people in America who is changing America".

It is noteworthy that the critical incidents mentioned by the 12 extraordinary adults with learning disabilities rarely mentioned their parents, spouses, partners or friends. Those individuals, who of course can be a source of support, simply were not mentioned. The people associated with critical incidents were teachers, teachers, and teachers. Henry Winkler got his "first break" in acting from his music teacher who expressed confidence in his skills. Jack Horner benefitted from the advocacy of his high school science teacher when trying to go to college with his less than impressive grades. Patricia Polacco had a "Eureka experience" with her junior high school English teacher Mr. Falker who helped her figure out who she was and what her talents were. Gaston Caperton and Terry Goodkind spoke of a high school English teachers who inspired them. Interestingly, this cluster of critical incidents stem from teachers who taught subjects that were a source of their academic struggles – reading and language.

Negative critical incidents also occurred in school that were recounted in emotionally-charged vivid detail. Imagine how painful was Chuck Close's embarrassment during his school years because of his poor memory, or Gaston Caperton's inability to perform in a round robin reading activity. They described these events as if they had happened yesterday. Despite all their accomplishments, it was all too easy for them to relate those agonizing moments from their past.

There are other interesting trends, both positive and negative, when investigating critical incidents. Neil Smith, while having a magical story of success in professional sports, does not identify anything in his sports career as a critical incident. Perhaps what he did came so naturally that it was perceived as "business as usual." The critical incident he did speak of was that of becoming a sports executive after his prolific sports career– a role that he never envisioned for himself.

Then there were what might best be described as incremental critical incidents. Jack Horner pointed out that there were critical incidents all along the way without any one really standing out. Even when he won the MacArthur Genius award, he said it had more of an effect on his father than on him. Gaston Caperton expressed the belief that his critical incidents were "evolutionary," adding to the idea that critical incidents do not have to be mega-events but smaller personal or professional successes that lead to others.

A number of critical incidents spoke to the issue of career. Perhaps the most gut-wrenching example of a critical incident was the story that Kendrick Meek told us about a "make it or break it" test he needed to pass to become a Florida State Policeman. If he did not pass, there would be profound consequences for his career choice. He would have to leave the state police academy. But he did pass. It is interesting that he chose this as a critical incident rather than his election to the U.S. Congress. Dr. Haseltine easily pointed out her most significant critical incident as the choice of her medical specialty, obstetrics, and gynecology– an event that ultimately launched her to prominence in the area of women's health. Even Diane Swonk viewed her first economics course as a critical event despite a less than satisfactory professor. That was, however, the very beginning of her brilliant career.

Chapter 11

TEACHERS: THE GOOD, THE BAD, AND THE UGLY

If the teacher can engage you, the power of wanting to learn pulls you along. If I hadn't had good teachers and people who engaged me in the power of knowledge, then I do not think I would have made it.
                              – Terry Goodkind, Best-Selling Author

Just as with critical events, teachers have had a great influence on these extraordinary adults – some good and some bad. It is easy to see the marked influence of Henry Winkler's high school music teacher leading him into acting, or Terry Goodkind's English teacher exciting him about literature. "She made me believe in myself," he says, " . . . that I could do what I wanted to do . . . be a writer." Without a doubt, Patricia Polacco's teacher, Mr. Falker, had such a profound effect on her that it has lasted for a lifetime.

There are other examples of how teachers made a difference. For our interview participants who had reading challenges, a teacher who could reach them in a "different way" helped greatly. Gaston Caperton recounted, "In eleventh grade I had a teacher that made Shakespeare come alive. It made F. Scott Fitzgerald and Hemingway come alive, too. And I was soaking this learning stuff up. I was interested, so I have always been a prolific reader". He continued by speaking more generally about good teachers. "For people like me where school is hard, a good teacher is really critical. If the teacher can engage you, the power of wanting to learn pulls you along. If I hadn't had good teachers and people who engaged me in the power of knowledge, then I do not think I would have made it." Terry Goodkind told us of his English composition teacher who talked to him about writing and gave him things to read. Years later, after he had achieved success with his novels, he tracked her down in California just to say thank you. Moreover, he dedicated one of his books to her.

Jack Horner spoke of a high school science teacher who helped him feel a sense of accomplishment despite his poor grades. Moreover, that teacher helped him pursue college training despite an overall borderline high school record. "I had this high school teacher. I was taking classes from him in Biology and failing. But he was head of the science fair, and I was winning all these science fairs. I had a lot of support from people like that."

Then there are examples of teachers' influence that that go far beyond the classroom. Patricia Polacco's junior high school teacher, Mr. Falker,, helped her come to grips with what she discovered was her learning disability and the variety of issues that resulted from it. She remembered quite vividly, "I didn't want anyone to know how stupid I was, most of all my teachers. . . . What they knew was that I appeared to be intelligent yet made mediocre grades and no one understood why. George Falker helped me, and that is when I realized he was a gay man. He, in my opinion, was the only one who could see the pain because he stood in front of a mirror like I did, bewildered and upset about being in a body when everybody says, "This is what you are supposed to be like," but you can't. He also knew the shame I did, for very different reasons. I think if he had not walked into my life at that time I would not be here. My two children would not exist. A teacher finds the key and is brave enough to walk up to a kid and say 'Look, I think I know something here, and you're not stupid, and I think I can help you.' They save lives, literally."

Neil Smith speaks particularly of a mentor-like special education teacher, Jean Pierre, he had in his public school in New Orleans. "I can look back at some of my teachers who are proud of me. And they say I worked with him. I helped him and I did extra things for him. They were sent for a reason. They were put in place to help kids. And as I went from junior high school to high school to college I just felt I had a special mentor for me in college . . . this gentleman."

Florence Haseltine also identifies a special education teacher as being very influential in her K-12 school experience. "The most important teacher was a special education teacher of mine about sixth or eighth grade. I would see her twice a week, mainly because of a lisp. She helped me with that and she also learned I could not read. She taught me speed reading. I learned to read about age 11 and went and got a book and started to recall, sort of overnight. She taught me the Evelyn Woods course. I do not know why but what she thought turned out to be really accurate. It turned out to be exceedingly helpful . . . particularly all I have to read for my job in medicine."

For Diane Swonk, the decision to become an economist came serendipitously from an entry level course taught by a noted economist and chair of the University of Michigan Economics Department. She describes him as a horrendous professor who was a wonderful economist serving at one time on the Federal Reserve Board. She admits, "I don't believe that I fell in love with economics under that professor. . . . It was just everything I had done up to then. It just clicked even though the professor was horrible. It was the easiest thing for me. I just kept going."

Then there are the negative experiences with teachers that are indelibly etched in the memories of some. Gavin Newsom describes the painful experience of round-robin reading not uncommon to classrooms in his day. "I remember being humiliated in my fifth grade class. My heart was pounding, I thought don't call on me, don't call on me to read that paragraph. And he does, and I will never forget. Everyone's starting to laugh at me because I couldn't even read a paragraph."

Perhaps one of the most painful experiences conveyed by any of these extraordinary adults came from Chuck Close. "My eighth grade teacher for whom I unfortunately had history, English and math – everything except art and music. She was really by-the-book. That was the first time I got straight D's. She couldn't fail me because I worked too hard. It was really devastating. She was my advisor in high school, and she told me I would never go to college and that I should go to a body and fender school or something like that. When I graduated the University of Washington, I had an unofficial transcript and sent it to her with a note saying 'I hope the next time you fail someone and say they cannot go to college remember me when I am in *Time* and *Newsweek.*' Then there is [person's name deleted] it is the only name I can remember – that [explicative]. I am a nonviolent person, lifelong pacifist, but if I got in an alley I'd run over her with my wheel chair, back and forth a couple of times."

What can be said that has not already been said of the teachers who have a profoundly positive effect on their students? The previous section on critical incidents has relevance for this section as well. It is not difficult to see the connection between critical events and memories of teachers that linger many years after leaving school. Those memories are not necessarily related to the content of the courses but often to the style and sensitivity of the teachers who taught them. How powerful is the interaction with a teacher who instills confidence in a student, confidence he or she never felt before, in any other class? Or an understanding of what the struggle feels like, thus fostering a unique kind of empathy? It seems the overriding message from these teachers was: Everything will be okay because you are okay. That validation is one of the tipping points that make a significant and positive difference. For students with learning disabilities, it lessens the pain of school and provides a *raison d'être* for being there.

The teachers who have been discussed by the people in this book are mostly teachers they had during their school-age years. That is noteworthy because all of them continued their studies in higher education in undergraduate school and beyond. This trend in responses points out where the influence of teachers might be the most important – when these students were most vulnerable. Thus, the teachers with whom they "connected" were a protective factor in their lives, the key ingredient of resilience. Often, the presence of positive or negative feelings about one's self is the difference between success and failure.

On the other hand, there are those teachers who are remembered for their lack of compassion, their harshness and negativity. What can be said about being in their classrooms the 180 days of an entire school year, day in and day out? Those teachers have a very "special" place in their memories of school. Chuck Close puts it all in perspective when recalling his eighth grade teacher. Low expectations, characterized by a suggested career in body and fender repair, were the best she saw for him. Luckily, he and his parents did not listen to her counsel. They saw other possibilities for him. Teachers like her need to be careful when predicting the future for their special needs students (or any student for that matter). They just might be listened to! It is sad to think how many students may have done just that. Moreover, what is viewed as optimal performance in eighth grade is only a snapshot in time. Chuck Close, who was not a stellar 14- year-old became a terrific 24-year-old at Yale and an even better 34-year-old as his stature and artistic reputation grew. Little has to be said about his legacy in the world of contemporary art at the age of 64.

All in all, there is no doubt that when one has a learning disability such as dyslexia, teachers who can foster a positive educational experience are invaluable. The teachers who are detrimental to the growth and development of their students need to realize how powerful their negative influence is. Certainly, it is difficult enough struggling with school without adding more to that burden.

Chapter 12

DISCLOSING THEIR LEARNING DISABILITIES

I know exactly when it happened. I will never forget it. I was a medical student sitting in the front row. . . . I was sitting in class and this professor starts to describe dyslexia and learning disabilities. And he described them right down the line and I yelled out, that's me! And the whole class clapped. 'Cause they knew it. So I was elated. I thought it was the greatest thing that ever happened to me. And I will never forget how I was suddenly relieved.
— Florence Haseltine, M.D., Ph.D., Physician and Scientist

The decision of going public about one's disability is very personal and quite private. It strikes to the heart of how one prefers to be viewed by others in myriad adult settings. Disclosure is very complex, and the decision to disclose learning disabilities or dyslexia can have both positive and negative outcomes. The person with learning disabilities such as dyslexia is very much in control of the information that is pertinent to disclosure of his disability. In essence, the individual himself manages this very personal, highly confidential information. Unlike the school-age years where students who are labeled "learning disabled" are typically tested, identified and placed in special education settings under the auspices of federal and state mandates, adults have the Shakespearean option of "to be or not to be" learning disabled or dyslexic because of its invisible nature. The choice to disclose (or not) is often measured in terms of the dynamics of employment, family, personal, social or leisure settings.

Disclosure can be a risky process. The way it is done can be likened to risk management. There are potential gains (some very great) when it works well. Relationships, whether personal or professional, are enhanced by greater understanding of behavior and performance. On the other hand, there are acceptable losses (choosing to keep the issue quiet) when the choice to disclose seems too risky. Not to disclose is a choice made to protect oneself from possible stereotypes, ostracism and negativity that marginalize one's daily routine. Often, those responses harken back to some uncomfortable and sometimes very painful school-age memories.

Learning about self-disclosure in the extraordinary adults we interviewed is interesting and important because it unearths a variety of issues and ideas that have not been uncovered through previous research. Without question, disclosure of learning difficulties by prominent individuals can do much to inspire others with similar problems, as well as help enlighten those working in the field of learning disabilities to positive life outcomes despite academic struggles. It can also expand our thinking about what people with dyslexia and other learning disabilities are capable of doing, thus shifting our focus away from a strictly deficit-driven model. Not long ago, there were few role models or exemplars of accomplishment to which school-age students could aspire. Now, because of disclosure, often in the form of speaking, there is proof that one can make it "in spite of the odds". The message is powerful and highly motivational, "I can be whoever I want to be despite having learning disabilities."

Not surprisingly, all the extraordinary adults we spoke with knew they had many challenges while in school because of a variety of learning problems. None indicated that they were placed in special education classes, and related quite vividly the obstacles they encountered in trying to learn and to "keep up." Small wonder that disclosure did not come during the school-age years, but rather only after they left school. However, in most cases these extraordinary adults came to realize they had what was called "learning disabilities" while in school, even prior to a formal diagnosis.

There are two examples of disclosure while in higher education settings. Dr. Haseltine related, "Oh, I know exactly when it happened. I will never forget it. I was a medical student sitting in the front row. . . . I was sitting in class paying attention and this professor starts to describe dyslexia and learning disabilities. And he described them right down the line and I yelled out, that's me! And the whole class clapped. 'Cause they knew it. So I was elated. I thought it was the greatest thing that ever happened to me. And I will never forget how I was suddenly relieved."

Kendrick Meek had a very different experience because of his mother's work as a legislator. His comfort in talking about his own learning disability stemmed from the inspiration he received from his mother's work. "My mom was in the (state) Senate at the time, and she went to the Congress. And at every level she was able to pass legislation to bring the education system in focus on kids with learning disabilities and learning difficulties. So then I started talking to the students at Florida A & M about the learning development center, and they started coming to the program. I spoke to them, counseled them and started speaking publicly."

Most of the individuals we interviewed disclosed their disability after success had come their way. Neil Smith never spoke about his learning disability while he was at Nebraska earning All-American football honors. It was only after he was in the pro ranks that he disclosed. "As a pro I felt like I was in the spotlight enough to know what people wanted to hear. It was something I had in me, and I could go [come] out because people look at you. They look at you like a superstar, and say, 'You are great at what you do, and you are one of the best. You won Super Bowls!'"

Patricia Polacco converted her disclosure experience into one of her most famous of the 60 children's books she has written. "The first time I disclosed was when I was an author. Disclosure came when I was talking at Ohio State University, making one of my 'speechie weechies.' For the first time I spilled out about what I am and from that standpoint of shame. It was a liberating force. Soon after my disclosure I wrote the book, *Thank You, Mr. Falker*".

Gaston Caperton first disclosed while he was serving as governor. He told us about a conversation about disclosure he had with then Governor Cain (of New Jersey) who is also reputed to be dyslexic. "We talked about it in a comfortable way. I was totally comfortable. I just never thought about doing it [disclosing] before. I didn't think anybody cared about it. I wasn't trying to hide anything. I sort of thought it was like having brown hair. It was just part of who I was and I moved on." He went on to relate how he first disclosed his learning disability in a public setting. "I did it when I was governor, at a public meeting. Every once in a while, particularly when I was home in West Virginia, people would come up to me and say my mother gave me an article when I was in sixth grade that you were learning disabled. It inspired me and I knew I could go to college."

Gavin Newsom related a story of how, as mayor of San Francisco, he first disclosed while speaking to school children. "The kids at the Armstrong [School] read that I mentioned it in passing, and they wrote a beautiful letter inviting me to their school. Then it became more public. The *Chronicle* did a front page story on my coming out with dyslexia and talking about it for the first time. Now I talk about it freely and openly." It should be noted that all three politicians in the group of extraordinary adults never spoke of their disclosure in negative terms. It also has never been used against them in a political contest.

Terry Goodkind disclosed his learning disability through reports that he shared with the media...He was very low-key about the issue of disclosure. "It's never been a big deal. I never had any sense of shame about it. It's hard for others to make a big deal out of it if you don't. I do not know anyone that has had a reaction other than, oh really, I'll be damned." Chuck Close related that the first time he disclosed publicly was when he spoke as an honoree at the Lab School for students with learning disabilities at American University in Washington, D.C. "I think it was the first actual time that I spoke publicly in front of a group. Now I virtually never speak without talking about it in almost any context. If I give a lecture in front of a school group or a university group, I always talk about it." Diane Swonk frames her initial disclosure moment in the context of being one of the relatively few women who are considered highly successful. "I guess it was in that *Forbes* article on *The Dyslexic CEO* with Chuck Schwab that I first talked to a reporter. I guess they didn't have enough women. So they ended up putting me in it". (Author's note: Of the five dyslexic prominent business leaders profiled in the *Forbes* article, Swonk was the only woman.)

Charles Schwab gave an interesting version of disclosure, emphasizing the role of terminology. "Well, coming out of the closet (as I call it) there was always an issue around the word dyslexia which I was never happy about. It really is a mysterious word to most people. And I really came to a conclusion, which is controversial in some ways. Learning difficulties or learning differences [are the terms] I like to use because I learn differently. And I always felt that way because I learn differently. I learned it doesn't mean you have dyslexia, you can't learn, you just learn differently. And so that was my own semantics of myself."

Interesting points arise out of their words. First, it took some time for the adults to disclose their learning disabilities after they experienced them in school. The first step of the disclosure process was receiving a diagnosis and a name for a perplexing condition they experienced every day of their lives during school or after leaving school. That diagnosis no doubt provided both a relief and an explanation. However, it is notable that no one disclosed until they were adults who already had laudable accomplishments in their careers. The exceptions are Florence Haseltine and Kendrick Meek, whose successes came later. Certainly it is easier to disclose one's learning disabilities when it comes as part of highly regarded work. The reaction "I'll be damned" shared by Terry Goodkind is quite telling. How much easier it must be to reveal learning disabilities amidst great success. Similarly, it is easier for the person hearing the disclosure to accept it from a person who has achieved extraordinary success.

What a difference being successful in adulthood makes, especially given the accomplishments and contributions of the individuals described in this book. In their early years, learning disabilities were a source of doubt and shame. The less their peers knew about the struggles associated with learning disabilities, the better. Surely, the invisibility factor helped, but the secret is difficult to keep with the omnipresent issues of academic performance and grading, teacher responses and expectations. One might wonder if any of the 12 people chronicled in this book would have voluntarily disclosed their learning challenges if they had not become so successful.

Just as there is a clear difference between the childhood and adult experience of learning disabilities, so too are there differences in the dynamics of disclosure at various life stages. Without question there are people with dyslexia and other learning disabilities who leave their labels behind when exiting school; it becomes emblematic of a time that may need to be "put away" and rarely revisited. On the other hand, perhaps the more successful one becomes, the more open one can become about having a disability. After all, isn't success the ultimate vindication? The notion of doing something a different way (their own way) and becoming successful allows disclosure without any residual negative feelings.

There is obviously less risk when people declare that they have learning disabilities such as dyslexia when they are successful. Their work speaks for itself and may counterbalance any negative consequences. Celebrity and adulation are constant reminders of their standing among their peers and in contemporary culture. Perhaps there is greater risk in disclosing one is learning disabled or dyslexic in the political arena. But that has never been an issue for Gaston Caperton, Gavin Newsom or Kendrick Meek. What becomes important with this freedom to disclose is the inspiration that it gives to others. Moreover, as role models they bring into focus the many positive things that are possible, in spite of having a learning disability. That seems to be the position of those described in this book. They have had a profound effect on people who aspire to pursue careers in the arts, literature, science, politics, and sports. They have provided an important foundation for a new era of opportunity for those who have learning problems, and not a moment too soon. A short 25 years ago, thinking about the prognosis for successful outcomes, high success and extraordinary success was less optimistic. Times certainly have changed– for the better.

Chapter 13

TECH SUPPORT

I'm introduced to words that I should have known in 9th grade, but because of my challenges . . . I still get on my computer and type the word in [using available dictionary or thesaurus] to get the full meaning of it.
— Kendrick Meek, Politician

A number of studies (including several by Marshall Raskind) have shown that technology can be of great value in helping people with learning disabilities compensate for their difficulties in the areas of reading, writing, math, listening, organization and memory. These technologies include word processors and speech recognition systems for writing, spell checkers for spelling, text-to-speech systems and books on tape/CD for reading, "talking" calculators for math, and personal data managers for organization and memory. These compensatory or "assistive" technologies often help individuals work around a problem by playing to their strengths. The goal is not to alleviate or fix deficits, but rather to bypass them. For example, optical character recognition systems with text-to-speech convert text on computer to speech enabling people with reading difficulties to convert printed text to spoken language. In this way, they can hear what is written rather than struggle to "break" the written code. Many people with dyslexia can understand the spoken word much more easily than the written word. Similarly, some people with learning disabilities in the area of writing find it easier to speak or dictate rather than write. In such cases, software that converts the spoken word to written text (speech recognition systems) may be helpful. It is interesting to note that some research has shown that technologies used to work around learning difficulties may, in some instances, also help to alleviate skill deficit. Although we did not ask our interviewees specifically about technology, several of them mentioned the impact technology has had on their lives. According to Florence Haseltine, "When the Macintosh computer came out, I bought the first one. I got the first spell check . . . and that changed my entire life overnight. The ability to type something, make a correction, and . . . not retype the whole page was the single biggest thing that ever happened to me." Diane Swonk made a no less dramatic statement about how technology impacted her life. "Something about the word processor, when I first got into it – the computer industry revolutionized my life. It made me a writer."

Congressman Meek spoke of using the computer to compensate for reading difficulties. "I'm introduced to words that I should have known in 9th grade, but because of my challenges," he says, "I still get on my computer and type the word in [using available dictionary or thesaurus] to get the full meaning of it." Terry Goodkind, like Florence Haseltine, spoke of how the computer helps him bypass spelling difficulties. ". . . I wanted to learn how to . . . write on a computer" he told us, ". . . to get around the fact that I can't spell, because computers had spell check and I thought . . . if I just learn how to use a computer I can get around that problem. So, you get around problems by finding the solution to it." Charles Schwab mentioned his use of Dictaphones to assist him with writing "way back when" as well as his enthusiasm for speech recognition systems that automatically convert speech to electronic text. Although they were not available when he was young, he says, "I love the books on tape. I listen to them all the time."

Although a number of these extraordinary individuals mentioned technology as a means of compensating for their difficulties, several of them did not. In fact, two indicated that they were not "big users" of technology. As is consistent with research on learning disabilities and assistive technology, what may be helpful to one individual may be inappropriate for another. The potential benefits of assistive technology for people with learning disabilities are dependent upon the interplay between the particular person, the task to be accomplished, the setting, and the specific technology. Nonetheless, based on what some of the participants in this study have said, it seems to make sense to consider technology as one possible strategy for dealing with learning problems.

Children growing up with learning disabilities today will likely have greater exposure and access to compensatory technologies than the extraordinary adults we interviewed. Hopefully, such opportunities will enable the next generation to bypass difficulties and accentuate strengths that will permit self-expressions at levels commensurate with their abilities and talents rather than their difficulties. Unfortunately, there are those who still view technology as a crutch for those with learning problems and believe that it will prevent them from learning the skills they need to succeed. Such thinking seems misguided. If Diane Swonk and Terry Goodkind did not have the benefits of word processing and spell checkers, would they have been able to compensate sufficiently to show their greatness? Of course, we cannot know, but reflecting on the exceptional talents and perseverance in these individuals the answer might certainly be yes. Even if the answer is yes, what personal cost to their self-esteem, time and energy would have occurred if they had to struggle continuously with the conventions of writing, possibly at the expense of detracting from the brilliance of their thinking. Research has shown us that for many people with learning disabilities, writing can be an anxiety-producing task. Yet, research also indicates that assistive technologies can significantly reduce apprehension in writing, as well as enhance the overall quality of content, grammar, punctuation and meaning.

It is also important to note that the very act of using compensatory technologies may in and of itself serve to alleviate specific learning difficulties. Research suggests that using technologies like word processors, spell checkers and speech recognition not only help people while they are using them, but that their written language abilities may show improvement even when the technologies are not being used. For example, consistent use of computer-based spell checkers may enable an individual to spell better even when they are writing with paper and pencil. Finally, the use of assistive technologies and instructional strategies to alleviate skill deficits are not mutually exclusive. There is no reason why a child struggling with reading couldn't, or shouldn't, be able to experience the joy of reading through audio books while also receiving the latest research-based instructional interventions for dyslexia. Shouldn't everyone, including those with dyslexia like Charles Schwab, know the joy of reading, albeit through an audio-book, rather than printed text?

Chapter 14

SPORTING CHANCE

In hindsight, the godsend for me was developing a strong aptitude for sports [primarily baseball, basketball]. . . . I don't think I would have been put in a position to have to start to believe in myself and start developing the self-confidence to apply myself academically had I not developed a sense of esteem because of success in sports.

— Gavin Newsom, Politician, Business Executive

Going back only a few decades, most people with learning disabilities were also thought to have coordination, motor and movement problems. It was not uncommon for professionals to equate learning disabilities with a child who also was awkward and had difficulty in sports. This may have been partly due to differences in definition and criteria used to determine learning disabilities four decades ago. Or perhaps it was the prevailing diagnostic and intervention models for learning difficulties –referred to as perceptual-motor– that reinforced this idea. However, this idea or myth was dispelled as Gold Medal Olympians known to have learning disabilities like diver Greg Louganis, decathlete Bruce Jenner, and runner/sprinter Carl Lewis achieved recognition. Other sports greats who had learning disabilities include race car driving champion Jackie Stewart, professional golfer John E. Morgan, and San Francisco 49ers quarterback Nate Davis.

Several of our interview subjects told us how their talent in sports provided an outlet, escape, or empowering experience that helped them counteract or buffer some of the negative experiences associated with having a learning difficulty. Perhaps, success in areas other than school, like sports, can help build self-esteem that may help steer someone on the road to positive life outcomes. According to Charles Schwab, "I think my early childhood success came in athletics. I was a very good, at least I thought I was, baseball player. And I loved playing all the athletic things, all the team things. So although I might not have been that good, but I thought I was pretty good . . . that was a great escape for me--baseball, basketball even." Eventually, it was his skill at golf that got him a scholarship to Stanford.

Governor Caperton explains, "I was a good athlete . . . I've always been a competitor . . . I knew when I was an athlete that I was a good leader, people followed me . . . I could inspire people. And so you kind of build on your own successes . . . you follow your strengths out there. You don't try to be something you're not."

In explaining how he found his niche, Gavin Newsom provided a poignant account of how sports helped him. "In hindsight, the godsend for me was developing a strong aptitude for sports [baseball, basketball, primarily]," he told us, "I don't think I would have been put in a position to have to start to believe in myself and start developing the self-confidence to apply myself academically had I not developed a sense of [self-] esteem because of success in sports. And, because of that, instead of just being a dumb student that was humiliated in Mr. Morris' 5th grade class when my heart is still pounding, please don't call me, please don't call me, to read that paragraph, and he does it and I'm standing up and I'll never forget it, you know I'm still there, physically can see it, everyone's starting to laugh at me because I couldn't even read that paragraph. I don't think I would have gotten through that, I think I would have had that struggle in perpetuity had it not been for sports and so I was able to excel in something that gave me confidence to then, just again, work harder to try to sort of re-apply myself."

Congressman Meek also spoke of sports, "I wouldn't say that I set academic goals, I was more of an athlete student, in school. Because I knew that's what I could conquer. I was an all county football player and . . . played basketball, . . . I was able to achieve there . . . and it was very difficult for me in school, . . . And, football allowed me to have an opportunity not only to conquer but to achieve and be recognized for that . . . achievement . . . was recruited by, quite a few universities . . . that wanted me to come play football".

Neil Smith's extraordinary achievements came in the realm of sports. "School was never up to par . . . [with] being an athlete because it was something I was more developed to do. You know I fell in with sports, at a young age, 5 years old. . . . it was something that I always wanted to do. I mean, I could do this all day and all night. . . . Just don't make me go before the class and read. So, in a sense, sports were my escape and I was good at it. . . . I would never brag, in any way but, you know, looking back, it's okay."

Although a number of the extraordinary adults in this study did appear to excel in sports, it would be misleading to give the impression that every one possessed such talent or found refuge in sports. It would also serve to establish a myth on the opposite end of the spectrum that all, or even most people with learning disabilities are superior athletes. In this project, only four out of 12 adults with learning problems mentioned that they had a talent or found "protection" in sports. In fact, Chuck Close emphasized his difficulties with athletics, "I couldn't hit a ball, I couldn't catch a ball, I couldn't throw a ball, I couldn't run. I had neurological problems my whole life . . . I couldn't keep up with my friends, I wasn't athletic, I wasn't a student. . . ." Particularly in the school-aged years, many people with learning difficulties don't find the opportunities for success and achievement. These years are often filled with a sense of frustration, failure, and negative feedback surrounding academic achievement. However, other individuals have been fortunate to find special talents and supporting environments in which to express and accentuate these abilities. There are those in our study, as well as many others with learning disabilities, who have found exceptional abilities in sports/athletics, abilities that have served to buffer the predominantly negative experiences and milieu of the school environment.

Although very few will have the highly exceptional athletic prowess of Neil Smith, there are those who may very well show ability in sports that, if not exceptional, at least may outshine their academic abilities. This athletic skill may serve to shield them against what can often be an onslaught of deficit-, rather than strength-oriented responses from both adults and peers surrounding the school experience. Early opportunities to experience success in areas other than academics may serve to counteract negative responses and help boost self-esteem, something that has often been diminished for many who struggle with learning problems. This is not a notion that emerges solely out of this study; other studies have also shown that sports or other areas of competence like art or music can go a long way in promoting positive life outcomes for people with learning problems. Unfortunately, we too often forget the need for individuals with learning disabilities to experience success, and the respect and acceptance that comes with it. There is no suggestion here that students with learning problems should only participate in activities at which they can succeed, or that instructional efforts to alleviate academic difficulties should be stopped. Rather, we should emphasize that perhaps more attention, or at least equal attention, should be paid to what a person with a learning disability can do well. We are reminded by another extraordinary individual with dyslexia from another one of our studies, someone who went on to become an award-winning environmental builder who lamented that, "people spent so much time, trying to fix what was wrong with me, that they never found out what was right . . . I was pulled out of classes so often to receive remedial reading instruction, that I never got to participate in history and art, the subjects I really loved and was good at." Hopefully, we can take heed of such insider voices and let them guide us in formulating strategies and approaches to foster positive life outcomes for people with learning difficulties.

Chapter 15

PAYING IT FORWARD

What's the value of life? Helping someone every day.
                – Neil Smith, Professional Football Player and Sports Executive

A theme that surfaced for all participants was a firm commitment to helping others. "Giving back" is crucial to their lives. Speaking about the purpose of life, Neil Smith commented, "What's the value of life? Helping someone every day." Their altruism takes many forms. In some instances, it is supporting others in the workplace. In speaking about helping a young colleague at work, Diane Swonk relates, "It is really an important thing to identify with people and touch all humanity." There were a number of instances in which these extraordinary results provided generous financial support to numerous causes and humanitarian efforts. Neil Smith heads an educational foundation aimed at helping children and parents. Charles Schwab established a foundation focusing on education, human services, and health. Others gave generously of their time in support of social service programs. Some chose the route of public service. As Congressman Meek stated, ". . . it was my learning difference and understanding that there are children in the classroom going through that . . . that drove me to write the constitutional amendment to limit class size in the state of Florida."

Still others give back through their art. Henry Winkler and Patricia Polacco wrote children's books dealing specifically with the struggles of having learning problems. All 12 openly share their stories of struggle and triumph with others, in many cases widely through print and broadcast media. Their audiences often are individuals experiencing the same kind of challenges. We also noted an apparent sensitivity to the struggle of others, particularly children. In some cases this was directed more toward children struggling with a variety of difficulties, but for the most part it included all children. Governor Caperton stated, "I'm always happy to talk to people and hope something I say will inspire them . . . anything I can do to help people." He explains how having learning disabilities may have contributed to his sensitivity to others, "I think you also have a compassion for people dealing with problems." Henry Winkler speaks poetically of talking to children, "And, what is amazing is that if you talk to a child and *acknowledge* the child, it's like watching a garden you watered grow in 30 seconds."

It is not clear why these individuals showed a strong sensitivity to others and a focused desire to help and give back. It is also not clear whether as a group, these individuals were more altruistic than those without learning disabilities. Perhaps it was their own struggles that sensitized them to the challenges of others, or it could be argued that their successes enabled them to devote time and money to help others. As Diane Swonk said, "Being able to help others has been really rewarding . . . it helps me heal from the times I was put down for the way I was thinking . . . or doing my work." It is obvious that there are highly successful individuals who don't give back to humanity as well as individuals with limited means who nevertheless offer more than their share. Although not all participants in this research made mention of the relationship between their struggles with learning disabilities, nine said that their desire to give back was prompted and fueled by the challenges they faced, particularly as children. Only one person in the study mentioned that her desire to give back was not directly related to her own struggles with learning problems, although she didn't discount the idea that it may have contributed to it.

Trying to determine the reasons behind the altruism of these extraordinary individuals is far beyond the scope of this study and the expertise of the authors. The roots of altruistic behavior have varied explanations. There are those who believe altruism is a learned phenomenon, while others believe it is "biologically programmed." There are also those who find its roots strictly in religious or spiritual grounds while still others view it as an outgrowth of multiple factors. Regardless of the reasons behind selfless behavior to promote the welfare of others, the individuals with learning difficulties in this study appeared to have it in abundance. Perhaps it is another characteristic that accompanies those individuals who have accomplished extraordinary things despite struggles and adversity. Perhaps it is a special talent or strength that needs to be recognized and nurtured. Of course, this is merely speculation and only future research will provide answers to such questions.

Chapter 16

TOO TIDY A TALE

The field of learning disabilities has historically sought to find commonalities in a category of individuals that is defined as being heterogeneous by nature. Research questions regarding individuals with dyslexia and other learning disabilities often include: How are these individuals alike? What do they have in common? How are their difficulties the same? How are their life paths similar? What are the subtypes of learning disabilities? These questions often revolve around the areas of academic achievement, cognition, memory, language and social/emotional development.

Although the answers to such questions can help to further our knowledge of the causes as well effective interventions such a focus may obscure the fact that persons with dyslexia and other learning disabilities are first and foremost people who display great diversity in their strengths, abilities, and challenges. Essentially, overemphasis on commonalities increases the risk of "telling too tidy a tale" about this group of extraordinarily successful individuals.

So while our analysis of the interviews of these extraordinary individuals did strive to search for common threads and themes in their lives, we must also temper this knowledge with the understanding that these individuals vary greatly in their abilities and life experiences. We must always keep in mind that their life journeys, as with all people, may be very different. There are many roads that lead to myriad places. Consequently, what may work for one person is not necessarily best for another.

Furthermore, what often appears, on the surface, to be a common denominator begins to show a difference upon deeper reflection. In reflecting upon the individuals in this book, we do find that all of them experienced academic difficulties of varying degrees, particularly in the area of reading throughout the school-age years. Yet these reading difficulties were not all the same; some were mild and others more severe. Even in the area of memory, Kendrick Meek and Neil Smith speak of having excellent recall, while others like Gavin Newsom believe his memory is less than optimal.

There are those individuals who seemed to have extraordinary talents that were there from the start– the artistic ability of Chuck Close and Patricia Polacco, the gifted acting of Henry Winkler, the athletic prowess of Neil Smith and the brilliance of Florence Haseltine. Yet others, such as Mayor Newsom, Governor Caperton and Congressman Kendrick Meek, parlayed their common sense, entrepreneurial talents and social skills into the world of politics after being very successful business people before they entered the political arena.

Mentors were important for Patricia Polacco in her ultimate life's work of story-telling. Similarly, Kendrick Meek had a mother who preceded him in Florida politics. But what of the late bloomers who became successful later in life? Writers Polacco and Goodkind did not begin their literary careers until later in their adult years, and Smith became a successful football executive after first being an NFL football player. Haseltine, Schwab and Swonk took more of a conventional approach and used their academic preparation to launch their stellar careers. Despite their learning disabilities, they went to very prestigious universities for their undergraduate and graduate work.

There is a startling commonality for some individuals in the group. Passionate interests were there from the start, and they have served them well in their adult lives, as evidenced by their accomplishments, notoriety and celebrity. Chuck Close and Jack Horner share much in common. They fell in love with their respective fields as youngsters. Learning disabilities during their school-age years imposed difficult challenges. Both had parents who were told that basic vocational education would be the best route for them. Fortunately, the "advice" of professionals was not followed and they became giants in their fields. They did it by "staying the course", getting through school as best they could and pursuing their passions. In essence, they became the people they hoped to become, even when their futures did not seem very bright.

While growing up, Diane Swonk and Charles Schwab had their "basic training" via practical experiences and incidental learning, primarily from their parents. Is it mere coincidence that Schwab's formative business experiences were in retail or that Swonk was a natural in her first economics course at the University of Michigan after spending her formative years in the back yard of Detroit's automotive industry?

Is it surprising that these individuals became extraordinarily successful? The honest answer is both yes and no. Success requires working hard, taking control, being self-aware, and capitalizing on opportunities. They have done that well, therefore the answer is yes. At the same time they have learning problems, so the answer could very well be no. Intuitively one would think it is more difficult to succeed when a learning disability such as dyslexia is in the mix. In the case of these 12 individuals, they found their "goodness of fit." In other words, they found their niches and have never looked back. With their high profiles in their respective fields we are all beneficiaries of their successes. They have made a difference in spite of the fact that there were many who thought they might be "too different" to reach great heights or contribute significantly to society.

Chapter 17

IN RETROSPECT: WISDOM ABOUT THEIR LEARNING DISABILITIES

Just because you learn differently does not mean you do not have greatness inside you.
— Henry Winkler, Actor, Director, Producer, Author

It's finding that inspiration, that sense of purpose, that passion that made me realize there was something inside me [without] limits.
— Gavin Newsom, Politician, Business Executive

Having heard the stories of their trials and tribulations, successes and challenges, it would be a missed opportunity not to elicit suggestions and recommendations from these extraordinary people. After all, although they succeeded in their own ways, their views can be applicable to other individuals with learning disabilities. One could make a case to cast aside the views and advice of these prominent figures since their extraordinary talents don't truly represent the average person with learning disabilities. It is nevertheless important to hear their words and consider that what worked for them may also apply to others who face many of the same challenges.

It is noteworthy that the suggestions and recommendations proffered are underpinned by a "can do" attitude. There is a lot of fight in the way they view the challenges of their learning disabilities. A defeatist thought is nowhere to be found. One simply does not hear a tone of resignation. On the contrary, there is persistence and resilience in their thinking. After all, how could they have achieved what they have achieved if their thinking was any different? As Diane Swonk so aptly put it, "I kept going when the going got rough, and I got beaten up. Part of having a disability is knowing how to pick yourself up, dust yourself off and learn from what just happened."

There is also an interesting theme of emphasizing what one does best and de-emphasizing that which is problematic. Moreover, it seems that their collective voices implore those with learning disabilities to "do it their way", within their own style and capabilities. Henry Winkler spoke right to that point, "Just because you learn differently does not mean you do not have greatness inside you. The fact of the matter is when you leave school is when you will meet your destiny." This thought is consistent with the thinking that it is only after one leaves school that one can really find one's niche. Some say just get out of school in one piece, then you can live the life you wish to have, because you are more in control as an adult. A highly successful adult with learning disabilities from another study aptly exclaimed, "Thankfully, I no longer have to dissect frogs. Tenth grade is way in my past." Certainly that was a past in which he had to be good at everything in a prescribed curriculum – math, foreign language, English literature, American history, etc.. Gerber, in a previous writing, described this as the "valedictorian complex" where one had to be good in every subject to succeed in high school. This secondary school experience is one not replicated in the beyond-school years, not even in higher education. Gaston Caperton summed up the differences between the school and beyond school years quite well: "You have more freedom to do things that you do well when you are in [adult] life than when you are in school. I often tell people the hardest thing is to get through school. . . . When you get out of school, things get better."

Moreover, what is part of the learning disabled experience in the early years might become something very important in later years. It is the uniqueness that one has that can be parlayed into opportunity. Diane Swonk put it so very well in saying, "Embrace your uniqueness because it's *your* uniqueness, it is not sameness that is going to define you. So embrace who you are because that is very important." She continues, "Don't let other people define you." Similarly, Chuck Close advises, "Don't let other people's goals become your goals." These words run contrary to the typical school experience, where the goals for students with learning difficulties are to become like the other students without disabilities.

The prevailing wisdom of the extraordinary adults interviewed implores those with learning disabilities not to listen to those who cry defeat (particularly during the school-age years) or who try to change the attributes that ultimately might lay the foundation for success later on in life. Gaston

Caperton went so far as to say, "The things that challenge you in school might be the biggest assets for what you will be doing one day."

There is a firm belief among a number of these extraordinary adults that finding one's passion facilitates a comfort level of interests and talents which forge a path to success. In fact, those who were interviewed generally believed that there cannot be success without passion. Mayor Newsom emphasized, "It's finding that inspiration, that sense of purpose, that passion that made me realize there was something inside me [without] limits." Their advice, directed to the school-age students with learning disabilities is varied and relates to non-academic suggestions for fostering success. "Pick something you want to do and do not worry whether it is important to someone else" complements the theme of doing it your own way. That idea is coupled with the notion of passion. "I find it essential to pursue something you have a lot of passion about," advises Charles Schwab. Jack Horner speaks of passion in offering suggestions to parents, "Let them do what they have a passion to do, what they want to do. Don't try to turn them into somebody different. They're not. Don't try to make them learn differently than they do. Just let them go, let them be creative."

It is not surprising that the theme of perseverance and in fact, what may even be described as a "fighting spirit," is inherent to the suggestions of those interviewed. Kendrick Meek said it well, "Never give up, never lose focus." Similarly, Neil Smith stresses, "I never gave up . . . I just refused." Diane Swonk expressed the same idea, "Learn from your mistakes. You need to be able to refocus and get back up –the persistence, that's really the most important lesson– you don't stop and you don't let other people take you down." In responding to a question regarding the factors responsible for her success, Patricia Polacco said, "Tenacity. Sticking to it when everything inside you is screaming give up." At the same time, she emphasizes that, when faced with obstacles, you may have to "redirect" your efforts. "I thought I could do it this way, but I guess I can't, so let me try this." Interesting, such flexibility in the face of adversity has been noted by Marshall Raskind in his studies of success attributes in people with learning disabilities. This seemed to be the overriding thought of Chuck Close when he said, "Do something over and over and do it each day. Even if it is a teeny little something, eventually you will have something. If you don't do anything you will never have anything. I say inspiration is for amateurs. The rest of us just show up and get to work because something in the process will occur, and it will open doors you never dreamed of, and things will happen. If you are sitting around waiting for inspiration it is never going to happen." Similarly, in explaining what he referred to as his "triangle of success," Henry Winkler emphasizes that both tenacity and preparation are crucial.

There is no doubt that the passion for their interests drives success, yet it is not without a cost. There is a lot of time and energy needed to fuel passion and drive success. Diane Swonk captures the cost of being successful that is universal, whether in school or in one's adult years: "Life is not going to be served to you on a silver platter. It's about attainment, not privilege. You learn attainment by having overcome obstacles. . . . That, in the end, makes you a leader. I think what is really important to understand is your challenges and your ability to overcome them makes you a problem solver."

When it comes to living with learning disabilities as an adult, the wisdom of Diane Swonk underscores the necessity to reframe learning disabilities as a given and not a "condition" that inhibits the adult experience. She has commented, "LD is as much a part of me as my eyes, my arms, my voice, my cadence . . . it is who I am. It is a part of me that I have integrated into myself rather than isolating it like it is a monkey on my back. It is much easier to go through life." Gaston Caperton's thought about having learning disabilities fits well with that of Diane Swonk. He advises others to "deal with LD knowing you have sensitivity to life and the determination for life. It will make you a better person if you have the right perspective about it."

Of course one can see the drive for success as these extraordinary adults with learning disabilities become cheerleaders for others. Terry Goodkind takes an approach to accomplishment that is consistent with the intra-individual differences that people with learning disabilities are known to have. "Everybody has his own level of learning," he points out, "Just figure out how to accomplish what you need to accomplish and move on. Just get it done. . . . Don't feel that you cannot do it. Just find out a way and just do it." Kendrick Meek sees the opportunity to only get better in adulthood. He advises that "It is never too late to improve." Moreover, some people take their whole life to get better." Self-motivation is their advice to adults with learning disabilities, as summed up by Neil Smith, "Take one day at a time. It will make you grow every day. Every day I want to learn something . . . I do not know." Overall, this approach rests on forging ahead despite one's learning disability. Gaston Caperton warns that you cannot use learning disabilities as an excuse. Moreover, Terry Goodkind adds that making a big issue out of dyslexia is not helpful.

Parents received advice to help them guide their children through the "learning disability experience." Florence Haseltine warns to do want you want to do and not worry about what others think. In fact, several of the adults interviewed have stated emphatically that one should not let others define what you *can* do or what you *should* do. Jack Horner advises, "Don't try to turn children into somebody different or even make them learn differently than they do." He believes that such an approach takes their creativity away. Similarly, Diane Swonk says, "Accept your kids, help them embrace who they are, and figure out what they can do and compensate in a way that is not hiding it."

Other extraordinary individuals in this study, stress the importance of fostering self-awareness and acceptance. Terry Goodkind emphasizes that "It's important that adults not make a child feel that they have this handicap in life and they must carry it around like a back pack. . . It's important to teach a kid that it's okay, you have this difficulty and here are some ways around it." Patricia Polacco tells parents, "Don't push them. Relax. Your kid is brilliant in many ways. . . . Give them something to hang their hat on, [so they can say] 'here is something I can do. . .' build their imaginations, keep their imaginations alive."

A general sense that came from all those we interviewed is that parents should never give up on their children. That powerful thought is consistent with the core of the resilience literature that identifies a "protective factor" (in this case, a parent) as being the difference between the dichotomies of success and failure, learned optimism and learned helplessness. Kendrick Meek says, have "the patience of Job." Gaston Caperton points out that having high expectations is critically important; a parent should "not ever give up, [but] just believe in them." That thought is echoed by Neil Smith, who is also a parent of a child with learning disabilities: "Stick with them and never give up on them. Every day do something for them to make their life better." All in all, Charles Schwab reminds us that encouragement and building confidence go a long way. Moreover, Patricia Polacco elaborates on the dynamics of encouragement when she says, "Instead of trying to improve on what you are mediocre at, which means you are going to be mildly less mediocre, find out what you really do well and pour energy into that. Dwell on what a child does well. Build confidence there." Henry Winkler strives to tell every child he meets, "You have greatness in you."

Both Neil Smith and Diane Swonk speak of a concept also found as a factor contributing to success in the research of both Paul Gerber and Marshall Raskind. Gerber refers to it as "reframing" while Marshall Raskind and his colleagues use the term "transformation." This phenomenon refers to the ability to reframe or transform the difficulties and struggles associated with learning disabilities into something positive. Neil Smith commented that people who have learning disabilities "Need to flip it . . . make it be something successful." Diane Swonk in elaborating on whether learning difficulties are a gift, said "I have evolved from it being a hindrance to being a gift."

EPILOGUE

The 12 individuals featured in this book are indeed remarkable. Yet they are representative of others with dyslexia and other learning disabilities who have accomplished amazing things. By design, this book focused on people with dyslexia and other learning disabilities in a variety of fields. We have written about CEO Charles Schwab and economist Diane Swonk, but we could just as easily have told the stories of John Chambers of Cisco Systems, Paul Orfalea, the founder of Kinkos, and the irrepressible entrepreneur Ted Turner, the force behind cable television in the United States.

Henry Winkler is representative of other actors with dyslexia and other learning disabilities, such as Orlando Bloom, Vince Vaughn, Danny Glover, Salma Hayek, and Kiera Knightly. Writers Patricia Polacco and Terry Goodkind are in good company with John Irving and John Grisham. So too is Neil Smith with baseball Hall of Famer Nolan Ryan, Formula One race car driver Sir Jackie Stewart, and gold medal U.S. Olympian diver Greg Louganis, decathlete Bruce Jenner and track star Carl Lewis. The stories of neurosurgeons Ben Carson and Fred Epstein, as well as Nobel laureate Dr. Baruj Benacerraf, leaders in their respective fields of medicine, could be told alongside that of Florence Haseltine. Chuck Close can easily be grouped with other famous artists like Robert Rauschenberg; politicians Kendrick Meek, Gavin Newsom and Gaston Caperton share dyslexia and other learning disabilities with Nelson Rockefeller, political strategist James Carville, and King Carl XVI Gustav of Sweden.

Without question there are many individuals with learning disabilities who are contributing handsomely to their respective fields of endeavor, although they may not have achieved the same level of public notoriety as the 12 individuals in this book. If one were to investigate other distinguished individuals with dyslexia and other learning disabilities, one would find names like Dr. William Gray, who did pioneering work in high definition television; Paul Grossman, federal government attorney specializing in civil rights issues pertaining to people with disabilities; David Willse, inventor of the health insurance model physicians preferred organization (PPO); Tom Sullivan, recently retired treasurer of the National Football League; John Corcoran, home builder and former member of the National Advisory Board member of the National Institute for Literacy; Delos Smith, former economist for the business-economics think tank, the Conference Board, headquartered in New York City; and Mike Tita, now retired, but long time chief problem-solver for the multinational 3M Corporation. And there are many, many others we can think of.

The point that should be made is that there are many individuals who are succeeding in spite of their learning disabilities, and in some instances, perhaps because of it. They have been able to succeed despite the odds, navigating the trials and tribulations of their learning difficulties. However, the same can be said of adults who may not have achieved "VIP" success status. Surely, success is subjective. Therefore, it is important to remember that tens of thousands of adults with dyslexia and other learning disabilities successfully contribute each day to their families, work groups and communities. Most have gone straight to work after high school. A few of them have gone on to study in college and some have even gone on to attain professional degrees. They, too, are examples of success, albeit not household names. They are all shining examples of succeeding in the face of adversity. They, too, deserve acclaim and admiration for what they have accomplished.

RECOMMENDED READING AND WORKS CITED

The following are materials from the professional and research literature that influenced our efforts in conceptualizing and writing this book. They also represent the body of work that helped frame the interview questions for the extraordinary adults with dyslexia and other learning disabilities.

BOOKS

Gerber, P. J. & Brown, D. S. (1997). *Learning disabilities and employment.* Austin, TX: PRO-ED.

Gerber, P. J., & Reiff, H. B. (1991). *Speaking for themselves: Ethnographic interviews of adults with learning disabilities.* Ann Arbor, MI: The University of Michigan Press.

Gerber, P. J. & Reiff, H. B. (1994). *Learning disabilities and adulthood.* Austin, TX: PRO-ED.

Roffman, A. J. (2000). *Meeting the challenge of learning disabilities in adulthood.* Baltimore: Paul Brookes.

Shaywitz, S. (2003). *Overcoming dyslexia.* New York: Vintage Books.

West, T. G. (1997). *In the mind's eye: Visual thinkers, gifted people with dyslexia and other learning difficulties, computer images and ironies of creativity.* New York: Prometheus Books.

ARTICLES

Baker, H. (1972). Famous people who have been handicapped: A critical analysis. Paper presented at the distinguished Lecture Series in Special Education and Rehabilitation, University of Southern California, Los Angeles, CA.

Gerber, P. J. (1993). Researching adults with learning disabilities from an adult development perspective. *Journal of Learning Disabilities, 27*, 6-9.

Gerber, P. J., Ginsberg, R., & Reiff, H. B. (1992). Identifying alterable patterns in employment success for highly successful adults with learning disabilities. *Journal of Learning Disabilities, 25*, 475- 487.

Gerber, P. J., & Price, L. A. (2006). Acceptable loss and potential gain: Self-disclosure and adults with learning disabilities. *Thalamus, 24,* 1, 49-55.

Goldberg, R. J., Higgins, E. L., Raskind, M. H., & Herman, K. L. (2003). Predictors of success in individuals with learning disabilities: A qualitative analysis of a 20- year longitudinal study. *Learning Disabilities Research and Practice, 18,* 4, 222-236.

Morris, B. (2002). The dyslexic ceo. *Fortune Magazine.* May 13, 54-70.

Raskind, M. H., Goldberg, R. J., Higgins, E. L., & Herman, K. L. (1999). Patterns of change and patterns of success in individuals with learning disabilities: Results from a twenty-year longitudinal study. *Learning Disabilities Research and Practice, 14*, 35-49.

Reiff, H. B., Gerber, P. J. & Ginsberg, R. (1997). *Exceeding expectations: Successful adults with learning disabilities.* Austin, TX: PRO-ED.

Rogan, L. & Hartman, L. (1976). A follow-up study of learning disabled children as adults. Final report. Project # 443CH60010, Grant #OEG-0-74-7453. Washington, DC: Bureau for the Education of the Handicapped, U. S. Department of Health, Education and Welfare.

Rogan, L. L. & Hartman, L. D. (1990). Adult outcomes of learning disabled students 10 years after initial follow-up. *Learning Disabilities Focus, 5*, 91-102.

Spekman, N. J., Goldberg, R. J., & Herman, K . L. (1992). Learning disabled children grow up: A search for factors related to success in the young adult years. *Learning Disabilities Research and Practice, 7*, 161-170.

ABOUT THE AUTHORS

Paul J. Gerber, Ph.D., received his doctorate in special education and school psychology at the University of Michigan in 1978. Before moving to Richmond he was a Professor of Education at the University of New Orleans and Associate Dean of the College of Education. Currently, he is a Professor in the Department of Special Education and Disability Policy in the School of Education at Virginia Commonwealth University in Richmond, Virginia. He also holds the Ruth Harris Professorship of Dyslexia Studies at Virginia Commonwealth University. Over the past 30 years he has researched and written extensively about post-school and lifespan issues for adults with learning disabilities, particularly employment. He has written numerous chapters and articles and co-authored four books in the area of adults with learning disabilities, one chosen as the top 20 resources for libraries by the American Library Association.

He has been a consultant to the U.S. Department of Education, the President's Committee for Employment of Persons with Disabilities (U.S. Department of Labor), the National Institute for Literacy, and the British Ministry of Health. Moreover, Dr. Gerber serves on a number of other editorial boards including the *Journal of Learning Disabilities, Learning Disability Quarterly, Remedial and Special Education,* and *Dyslexia: An International Journal of Research and Practice.* He is past editor of *Thalamus,* the journal of the International Academy for Research in Learning Disabilities. Fellowships that Dr. Gerber has been awarded are from the World Rehabilitation Fund and twice from the Project for the Study of Adult Learning (Illinois State University). He has won numerous awards including the Outstanding Researcher Award from the Virginia Council for Learning Disabilities, the Outstanding Paper Award from the Virginia Educational

Research Association, the Distinguished Paper Award from the Consortium of State and Regional Research Associations of the American Educational Research Association, and the Excellence Award at the Virginia Commonwealth University School of Education. He has given numerous keynote speeches and national and international presentations. Of note are the William M. Cruickshank Memorial Lecture for the International Academy for Research in Learning Disabilities and the Distinguished Lecture for the 50th Anniversary of the Marianne Frostig Center in Pasadena, California.

Marshall H. Raskind, Ph.D., Dr. Raskind has a Ph.D. in Education, with a focus on learning disabilities from Claremont Graduate School. He is former Director of Research and Special Projects at the Charles and Helen Schwab Foundation in San Francisco. Immediately prior to his position at the Foundation, he served as Director of Research at the Frostig Center in Pasadena, California. He is former head of the California State University, Northridge Learning Disability Program and Computer Access Lab and has also served on the faculty of Claremont Graduate School. He has been a consulting editor to the *Journal of Learning Disabilities, Learning Disability Quarterly, Annals of Dyslexia,* the *Journal of Special Education Technology*; and *Intervention in School and Clinic.* Dr. Raskind is a Fellow and past Vice President of the International Academy for Research in Learning Disabilities, a past member of the Research Committee of the Council for Learning Disabilities, and a former member of the Professional Advisory Board of the National Center for Learning Disabilities.

His research interests are in the areas of learning disabilities across the lifespan, factors predictive of "life success," and assistive technology. Most recently, he has directed his attention toward the impact of online social networking on children with learning disabilities and ADHD. Dr. Raskind is a frequent presenter at international learning disability conferences and is the author of numerous professional publications on learning disabilities. His research has been cited in the media, including *The New York Times, Fortune Magazine, Time Magazine,* and MSNBC.

INDEX

A

Abraham, 12
academic difficulties, 71, 75
academic performance, 63
access, 7, 20, 66
accommodation, xviii
accounting, xviii, 35
adaptability, xviii, 24
ADHD, 90
adjustment, xvi, xvii, 29
adulthood, xiv, xv, xvi, xix, 21, 24, 25, 28,
   29, 30, 31, 34, 45, 63, 82, 87
adults, ix, xiv, xv, xvi, xvii, xix, 1, 5, 18, 21,
   23, 24, 27, 29, 30, 31, 33, 34, 42, 45, 47,
   49, 51, 55, 57, 59, 60, 61, 62, 66, 71, 80,
   81, 82, 83, 86, 87, 88, 89
advocacy, 11, 52
African-American, ix, 10
age, 6, 7, 11, 12, 22, 27, 34, 36, 49, 50, 56,
   58, 59, 60, 70, 76, 80, 81
altruism, 73, 74
altruistic behavior, 74
American culture, 5
American Educational Research
   Association, 90
Americans with Disabilities Act, xix
anxiety, 67
aptitude, 41, 69, 70
arithmetic, xv

artery, 7
assets, 12, 45, 81
assistive technology, 66, 90
athletes, 5, 71
attitudes, xviii
attribution, 30
autonomy, 29

B

bankers, xvii
banks, 14
barriers, 20
basic research, xvii
behaviors, xiii, xviii, 40, 43
Belgium, 6
beneficiaries, 77
benefits, 29, 67
bias, 8
blame, 27
blueprint, 37
brain, 39, 41
broadcast media, 73
business model, 12

C

cable television, 85
case study(ies), 49, 50
Catholic school, 12

central nervous system, xiii
cerebral palsy, 15
certificate, 11
challenges, ix, x, xv, xvi, xviii, xix, 1, 3, 11, 12, 15, 20, 21, 23, 24, 25, 27, 30, 31, 36, 41, 42, 45, 47, 50, 55, 60, 63, 65, 66, 73, 74, 75, 76, 79, 82
chaos, 23, 35
Chicago, 6, 14
childhood, 24, 26, 29, 30, 31, 34, 63, 69
children, ix, xi, xv, xix, 2, 11, 13, 23, 25, 35, 37, 56, 61, 73, 74, 82, 83, 88, 90
China, 21
citizens, 1
city(ies), 1, 2, 3, 6, 13, 14, 34, 51, 86
civil rights, 86
clarity, 22, 30, 35
class size, 10, 73
classes, 56, 60, 72
classroom, xiv, xv, 5, 56, 73
clients, 12
clinical trials, 8
CNN, x
cognition, 75
cognitive abilities, xiv, 47
cognitive processing, 21
cognitive style, 47
colleges, 6
color, 18
commercial, 15
common sense, 76
community(ies), xvi, xvii, 12, 86
compassion, 39, 58, 74
complement, xviii
complexity, 48
composition, 55
computer, 22, 65, 66, 67, 87
configuration, 7
Congress, 2, 10, 52, 60
Congressional Budget Office, 14
constituents, 2
constitutional amendment, 73
consulting, 90
controversial, xix, 62
conversations, 18

coordination, 69
cost, 67, 82
counsel, 58
counterbalance, 63
creative process, 46
creativity, xvii, xviii, 45, 47, 83, 87
critical analysis, 88
criticism, 34
cues, 23
cultural differences, xiii
culture, 63
curriculum, 25, 80

D

daily living, xvi, 21
danger, 47
decoding, xiv
deficit, xiv, xvi, xix, 60, 65, 71
Democratic Party, ix
Department of Education, xiv, 89
deprivation, 25
depth, xvii
destiny, 80
dinosaur egg, 9
dinosaurs, 2, 9, 10, 36, 47
disability, ix, xiii, xiv, xviii, xix, 1, 5, 8, 9, 10, 11, 13, 17, 18, 19, 31, 39, 40, 41, 42, 43, 45, 46, 48, 50, 51, 56, 58, 59, 60, 61, 62, 63, 72, 77, 80, 82, 90
disaster, 40
disclosure, 59, 60, 61, 62, 63, 88
diversity, 17, 19, 75
DNA, 47
draft, 13
dream, 34
dyslexia, ix, x, xiii, xiv, xv, xvi, 1, 3, 5, 7, 9, 10, 14, 15, 17, 18, 19, 22, 24, 30, 33, 40, 42, 43, 46, 51, 58, 59, 60, 61, 62, 63, 65, 67, 72, 75, 77, 82, 85, 86, 87

E

economic development, 5

economic policy, 2
economics, 14, 35, 42, 53, 57, 76, 86
education, xix, 5, 6, 8, 13, 27, 56, 61, 73
educational career, 11
educational experience, 28, 58
educational settings, 17
educational system, 5
egg, 9
elders, 11
election, ix, 52
elementary school, xv
emotional problems, xiv
empathy, 39, 58
employees, 11, 12
employment, xiv, xvi, 21, 51, 59, 87, 88, 89
encouragement, 83
endocrinology, 8
energy, 48, 67, 82, 83
entrepreneurs, xvii
environment, 71
environments, 33, 71
epilepsy, 15
evidence, ix, xix, 9, 40
evolution, 47
exercise, 2
expertise, x, 8, 36, 74
exposure, 66

F

fairness, xix
faith, 49
families, 24, 86
fantasy, 3, 7
fantasy novel, 7
federal government, 3, 8, 86
federal law, xix
Federal Reserve, 14
Federal Reserve Board, 57
feelings, 58, 63
fertilization, 8
fibroids, 50
films, 9
financial, 1
financial failure, 11

financial support, 73
fine arts, 37
flexibility, 18, 81
football, 10, 13, 36, 51, 61, 70, 73, 76, 86
force, 22, 41, 61, 85
foreign language, 80
formal education, 51
France, 6
franchise, 51
freedom, 63, 80
funding, xi, 8, 17, 19

G

genus, 9, 34
geology, 9, 27, 34
gifted, 36, 76, 87
goal-setting, xvii
God, 34, 41
governor, 5, 35, 45, 61
grades, 34, 49, 52, 56
grading, 63
grass, 10
growth, xiv, 11, 21, 23, 58

H

hair, 61
health, 3, 8, 13, 53, 73
health insurance, 86
high school, 9, 10, 28, 49, 52, 55, 56, 57, 80, 86
higher education, 3, 27, 58, 60, 80
history, xvi, 8, 11, 37, 57, 72, 80
hotel, 2
house, 2
House of Representatives, 10
human, xviii, 7, 13, 73
human development, xv
Hungary, 6
hunting, 9
Hurricane Katrina, 13

I

icon, 36
identity, 8
idiosyncratic, 46
images, 87
imagination, 2
immigrants, 14
in vitro, 8
in vitro fertilization, 8
individual differences, 82
individuals, ix, x, xiv, xvi, xvii, xix, 3, 5, 17, 18, 19, 20, 24, 27, 31, 40, 42, 43, 47, 51, 60, 61, 63, 65, 66, 67, 71, 73, 74, 75, 76, 77, 79, 83, 85, 86, 88
industry, 14, 66, 76
ingredients, 45
injury, 11
intellect, 37
intelligence, xiv, xv, 30
intervention, 26, 69
investment, 13, 36
investors, 1, 48
issues, xiv, 1, 3, 18, 19, 21, 24, 26, 27, 29, 40, 43, 56, 60, 63, 86, 89

J

Japan, 21
junior high school, 11, 52, 56

K

kindergarten, 9

L

lack of confidence, 30
later life, 24
laws, xix, 8
lead, xviii, 36, 37, 39, 52, 75
leadership, 3, 5
learned helplessness, 28, 47, 83

learners, 19
learning difficulties, xiii, xiv, xv, xviii, 3, 37, 40, 43, 45, 47, 60, 61, 65, 67, 69, 71, 72, 74, 80, 84, 86, 87
learning disabilities, ix, x, xiii, xiv, xv, xvi, xvii, xviii, xix, 1, 2, 3, 5, 11, 12, 17, 18, 19, 20, 21, 23, 24, 25, 27, 29, 30, 31, 33, 39, 40, 41, 42, 43, 45, 46, 47, 49, 51, 58, 59, 60, 61, 62, 63, 65, 66, 69, 71, 74, 75, 76, 79, 80, 81, 82, 83, 85, 86, 87, 88, 89, 90
legal protection, 17
legislation, xiii, 1, 17, 19, 61
leisure, xvi, 21, 59
life experiences, 19, 75
lifetime, 36, 55
light, 25
longitudinal study, 88
love, v, 26, 51, 57, 66, 76
lying, 34

M

man, x, 2, 41, 56
management, 36
materials, 87
mathematics, 9, 12, 51
matter, 33, 37, 47, 58, 80
measurement, 36
media, ix, 62, 90
medical, 30, 50, 52, 59, 60
medical care, 8, 36
medical history, 8
medicine, 50, 57, 85
membership, 6
memory, 21, 23, 33, 34, 39, 52, 65, 75, 76
mental retardation, xiii
mentor, 56
military, 9
mission, xiv
models, xix, 60, 63, 69
mole, 30
Mongolia, 2
Montana, 9, 27, 34, 36
motivation, ix, xvi, 28, 33, 36, 47, 49, 82

multinational corporations, xvii
multiple factors, 74
museums, 6, 11
music, 39, 49, 52, 55, 57, 71

N

National Institutes of Health, xiv, 17
NATO, 10
negative consequences, 63
negative experiences, 57, 69, 71
negative outcomes, xviii, 59
negativity, 58, 60
New England, 40
next generation, 66
nuisance, 21

O

obstacles, 23, 46, 60, 81, 82
oil, 34
opportunities, 37, 66, 71, 77
optimal performance, 58
optimism, 83

P

pain, 50, 56, 58
paints, 7
paleontological investigation, 2
paleontology, 9, 22, 27
parents, ix, xv, xix, 11, 35, 36, 51, 58, 73, 76, 81, 83
participants, xviii, 55, 66, 73, 74
patents, 8
permit, 66
perseverance, xviii, 3, 67, 81
personality, 19
persons with disabilities, xix, 8
photorealist painter, 6
phylum, 34
physicians, 86
playing, 34, 65, 70
pleasure, 50

polar, 30
police, 51, 52
policy, 3
politics, 10, 11, 63, 76
population, xvi, xvii, 40
portraits, 2, 6, 7, 33, 42
positive relationship, xiv
potential benefits, 66
poverty, 13
preparation, iv, 76, 82
president, ix, 6, 11, 14, 37, 89
prevention, 13
problem-solver, 86
problem-solving, xviii, 45, 46, 48
problem-solving skills, 47
professionals, xix, 69, 76
profit, 6
prognosis, 63
project, xi, 71
protection, 71
prototypes, 28
public policy, 8
public schools, 10
public service, 73

Q

quarterback, 69
questioning, 30

R

race, 10, 69, 85
radar, 51
reading, xiii, xiv, xv, 9, 11, 12, 13, 17, 19, 22, 24, 25, 26, 27, 34, 36, 41, 42, 51, 52, 55, 56, 57, 65, 66, 67, 72, 75
reading comprehension, xiv
reading difficulties, 65, 66, 76
real estate, 11
reality, 8, 18, 48, 51
reasoning, xiii
recall, 56, 76
recalling, 58

recognition, 5, 65, 66, 67, 69
recommendations, 79
recreation, 21
reform, 11
Rehabilitation Act, xix
relevance, 48, 57
relief, 62
repair, 58
reputation, 58
requirements, 25
resilience, xviii, xix, 58, 79, 83
resources, 89
retail, 48, 76
rights, 7
risk, xix, 1, 59, 63, 75
risk management, 59
root, 22
roots, 10, 74
rules, 22

S

scholarship, 11, 70
Scholastic Aptitude Test, 6
school, xi, xv, 6, 7, 8, 9, 10, 14, 21, 22, 23,
    25, 26, 27, 29, 30, 34, 40, 49, 50, 52, 55,
    56, 57, 58, 59, 60, 61, 62, 63, 69, 70, 71,
    76, 80, 81, 82, 89
school achievement, 30
school psychology, 89
science, 11, 12, 26, 27, 36, 48, 52, 56, 63
scope, 74
security, 10
selective memory, 23
self-awareness, xviii, 31, 35, 83
self-concept, 17
self-confidence, 15, 42, 69, 70
self-esteem, 27, 67, 69, 71
self-expression, 66
sellers, 7
semantics, 62
Senate, 10, 60
sensitivity, 57, 73, 74, 82
September 11, 47
services, 13, 17, 19, 20, 73

shame, 56, 61, 62, 63
shape, 43, 49
showing, 12
signs, ix
silver, 82
social network, 90
social perception, xiii
social relations, 21
social relationships, 21
social skills, 76
social support, xvii, xviii
society, 77
software, 65
solution, 46, 49, 50, 66
spatial ability, 40
special education, xix, 56, 59, 60, 89
species, 34
species of dinosaurs, 9
speculation, 74
speech, 41, 65, 66, 67
spelling, xiv, 11, 22, 34, 65, 66
spending, 76
stars, 15
state, 5, 6, 10, 11, 23, 37, 52, 59, 60, 73
states, 1, 14, 18
statistics, 23
stereotypes, 60
stock, 48
storytelling, 11, 12
stress, 83
style, 19, 36, 42, 48, 57, 80
subgroups, xvi
Sun, 14
Super Bowl, 2, 13, 31, 61
support staff, 24
survivors, 28
Sweden, 85
synthesis, 42

T

talent, 11, 12, 34, 36, 37, 40, 69, 71, 74
teachers, xv, xix, 26, 27, 33, 34, 49, 50, 52,
    55, 56, 57, 58
teams, 13

technician, 9
technology(ies), 5, 65, 66, 67
teens, xv
teeth, 34
tenure, 5
textbook, 22
thesaurus, 65, 66
thoughts, 3, 17, 18, 29, 42, 46, 49
torture, 26
training, 8, 12, 30, 50, 56, 76
traits, 40
trajectory, 36
transformation, 83
traumatic events, 45, 47
treatment, xix
twist, 30

U

U.S. Department of Labor, 89
unemotional likenesses, 7
unidentified people, 7
United States, ix, 3, 6, 10, 85
universities, 6, 70, 76

V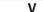

validation, 58
Vice President, 14, 90

videos, 1
vision, 2, 27, 39, 40
vocabulary, xiv
vocational education, 27, 76
vote, 2, 11

W

war, 36
war years, 36
Washington, 2, 6, 8, 34, 57, 62, 88
water, 25, 47
weakness, xviii
wealth, 13
welfare, 74
wildlife, 7
wood, 26
word processing, 67
word recognition, xiv
workers, 36
workplace, 36, 73
World Trade Center, 45, 47
worldwide, 1
worry, xv, 81, 82

Y

Yale University, 6, 7, 15, 34